CAN YOU IDENTIFY THIS PERSON?

When you were in school, you were always the class clown. At the beginning of a new school year, the other students were thrilled to see that you were in their class. They knew that with your practical jokes, wild bird calls, hilarious remarks, and impetuous antics, there would never be a dull moment.

Chances are, this is the baby in the family . . . just as it's a good bet the class president is first born. And "one of the gang," "just plain Jane," or "good old Bill" is the middle child.

Find out why and what it means for the rest of your life in . . .

THE BIRTH ORDER BOOK

"Dr. Leman tells poignant stories of his own experiences which match so many of those of his readers. . . . You want to keep his book near at hand!"
—*Orangeburg Times and Democrat*

"Entertaining and enlightening . . . offers down-to-earth tips on making your birth order work for you."
—*Christianity Today*

"Your birth order molds your personality. . . . Here's how to use it to get the most out of life."
—*The National Enquirer*

by Dr. Kevin Leman

MAKING CHILDREN MIND WITHOUT LOSING YOURS
THE BIRTH ORDER BOOK
BONKERS

THE
BIRTH
ORDER
BOOK

WHY YOU ARE
THE WAY YOU ARE

Dr. Kevin Leman

A DELL BOOK

Published by
Dell Publishing Co., Inc.
1 Dag Hammarskjold Plaza
New York, New York 10017

Dell ® TM 681510, Dell Publishing Co., Inc.

Reprinted by arrangement with Fleming H. Revell Company

ISBN: 0–440–10559–5

Printed in the United States of America

May 1987

10 9 8 7 6 5 4 3 2 1

WFH

To my first-born,
lovable perfectionist, Holly.
Your creativity, sense of fair play,
love for God,
and sensitivity to others
make me proud to be your dad.
I love you very much.

Contents

Part Four

Birth Order and Marriage: Some Better, Some Worse

Part Five

Birth Order and Parenting: Never Treat Them All the Same

Part One

What Is Birth Order . . . and Should Anyone Care?

Absolutely! Your birth order—whether you were born first, second, or later in your family—has a powerful influence on the kind of person you will be, the kind of person you will marry, the type of occupation you will choose—even the kind of parent you will be. In these first two chapters you will learn . . .

- the major characteristics of your birth order
- what first-born children have in common with outer space
- why the babies of the family are often show-offs
- how to pick the first borns in any crowd

- how the number of years between children creates different families within the family
- how a second born can take over from the oldest child
- the great danger in rearing an only child
- the child in your family you are most likely to favor

Chapter One

Birth Order?
Is That Like Astrology?

Whenever I mention "birth order" during a seminar or a counseling session, I'm often met with the same question: "Birth order—is that like astrology?"

And they often add, "Are you Taurus or Capricorn?"

Resisting the temptation to say, "No, I'm into pork bellies," I kindly reply, "Birth order has nothing to do with astrology, but it definitely affects your personality, whom you marry, your children, your occupational choice, and even how well you get along with God."

My questioner usually still looks skeptical, so I explain that we've known about birth order since the turn of the century, but it hasn't been given much serious consideration and study until the last twenty-five years. Now there are all kinds of books, journals, and research papers on the subject. You can get very detailed about birth order if you want, but to keep things simple in this book we will talk about three main birth order positions:

The eldest (and along with them the "only" borns)

The second (or middle-born) children

The babies (last born—the youngest)

This Is Only a Test

To start you off on what birth order is all about, let's take a little quiz. Which of the following lists of personality traits fits you the best? (You don't have to be *everything* on the list, but pick the list that has the most items that relate fairly well to you and your lifestyle.)

A. perfectionistic, reliable, conscientious, list maker, well organized, critical, serious, scholarly

B. mediator, fewest pictures in the family photo album, avoids conflict, independent, extreme loyalty to the peer group, many friends, a maverick

C. manipulative, charming, blames others, shows off, people person, good salesperson, precocious, engaging

You probably noted that I made it rather easy by listing traits of the oldest right on down to the youngest. If you picked list A, it's a good bet you are the first born in the family. If you picked list B, chances are you are a middle child (second born of three children, or possibly third born of four). If you related best to list C, it's likely you are the baby in the family and somebody had to buy this book for you. (I like to have a little fun with the babies of the family because I'm one myself, but more on that later.)

Notice, in each case I said something like "Good bet" or "Chances are." I don't have any strange supernatural powers when it comes to picking the birth order of any person, but there is an awful lot of research and plain old "law of averages" odds on my side. Just for fun, when conducting family life seminars around the country, I take a quick look around and spot ten people who I believe are first-born or only-born children. I go entirely by their physical appearance. These are the folks who look as if they've stepped off the cover of *Glamour* magazine or out of an ad for the *Wall Street Journal.* They're easy to spot. Every hair is in place and they are color coordinated from head to toe. I usually hit nine out of ten, often ten out of ten.

Some people in the audience start suspecting they have wandered into a performance by "Merlin the Magnificent" by mistake, but of course that's not true. There is, however, something to birth order because the odds definitely prove it out. It doesn't explain everything about human behavior—no personality test or system can—but it does give us many clues about why people *are* the way they *are*.

As a practicing psychologist, I have used my

15

training and research in birth order as a useful tool in helping people turn their lives around. Birth order information helps Mary understand why John is always so picky, and John gains insight into Mary's "little girl" ways, which are driving him more bonkers by the day. Birth order helps Mom and Dad get a handle on why ten-year-old Buford can go through life oblivious to his open fly and C+ average, while thirteen-year-old sister Hortense has straight *A*s and a good start on an ulcer.

What Do First Borns and Outer Space Have in Common?

Very little, actually; it's usually the babies of the family who qualify for "space cadet." But birth order continues to be revealing when you look at who's in what occupation. Of the first twenty-three astronauts sent into outer space, twenty-one were first borns or only children. In fact, all seven astronauts in the original Mercury program were first borns in their families.[1]

Research psychologists have come up with substantial evidence that shows first borns as more highly motivated to achieve than their younger brothers and sisters. A much greater proportion of first borns wind up in "high achievement" professions such as science, medicine, or law. You'll also find a greater number of first borns among accountants, bookkeepers, executive secretaries, engineers, and, in recent years, people whose jobs involve computers. First borns typically go for anything that takes precision, strong powers of concentration, and dogged mental discipline.[2]

I served for several years as Assistant Dean of Students at the University of Arizona and once asked a leading faculty member of the College of Architecture if he had ever paid any attention to where the college's faculty members came from as far as birth order was concerned. He gave me a blank stare and said, "I really have to run, Kevin."

It was probably a good six months before he stopped me on campus one day and said, "Say, do you remember that crazy question you asked me about where our architectural faculty came from? I finally decided to take an informal poll and found that almost every one of our faculty is either a first-born male or the only child in the family."

That was an eye-opener for my friend, but for me it only confirmed a basic birth order principle: people who like structure and order have a tendency to enter professions that are rather exacting. Architecture is one of those professions that pay off on being "perfect."

It's also fascinating to compare birth orders in the media. Newspaper and magazine reporters —those who write for a living—tend to be first

17

borns. Announcers and anchorpersons on radio and television tend to be later born. You could probably make a very good guess that your zany weatherman on the six o'clock news is the baby in the family. He's a performer, a showman. He's the guy who can make a drizzle seem funny. Youngest children in the family are often found in the professions that require the ability to be "on stage" and to perform.

The Leman Tribe and How We Grew

To give you a quick look at the three "typical" birth order positions, bear with me while I introduce you to the family I grew up in. (You'll meet my own family, wife Sande, daughters Holly and Krissy, and son Kevin II a little later.) Mom and Dad Leman had three children:

Sally—first born
John, Jr. (Jack)—middle child, born three years later
Kevin ("Baby Cub")—born five years after Jack

I'll explain the "Cub" business later because it remains my nickname to this day. But first a look at my sister, Sally, a classic first born who lives in a small town in western New York. I usually take my wife and children to visit Sally's immaculate house just about every summer vacation, and the first thing we all notice as we come through the front door is the *clear vinyl runner* which leads to every room in the house. The message is loud and clear: "Thou shalt not walk on the blue carpet, except where absolutely necessary."

Sally is the one who has butterflies at least two days before giving a small dinner party. Bigger dinner parties cause butterflies for a week or ten days. Sally's rule of thumb seems to be: "The bigger the dinner, the bigger the butterflies!" Of course, everything must be color coordinated: the napkins match the napkin holders, which match the decor of the formal dining room, which matches her husband's eyes. If possible, Sally would iron the "Welcome" mat.

No one in the Leman clan will forget the time we all gathered in the Sierra Nevada mountains for a camping trip. We had a terrific day in the great outdoors and by ten o'clock that night everyone was ready for the sleeping bags. At that altitude it would drop to fifty degrees and below and most of us planned to sleep in our jeans, sweat shirts, and whatever camping clothes we had brought along.

Not Sally. She came out of her tent to say good night, attired in her nightie and negligee, and couldn't figure out why we all dissolved in laughter. But why not a negligee on a camping trip when you are a former home economics teacher turned preschool director? Why not add a little class to the campsite when you are creative, artistic, and neat about everything you do?

When Sally does anything, she does it right. All her life she has been confident, scholarly, well liked (she was a cheerleader in high school) —a National Honor Society type all the way.

My brother, Jack, was born second and, as with a lot of middle children, it is a bit more difficult to pin down his precise personality traits. For one thing, the second child is known for going in exactly the opposite direction from the first born in the family. But Sally was such an all-American type—cheerleader, good student, popular, etc., etc.—that to go in a completely different direction would have taken Jack to the pool hall and perhaps reform school.

In high school Jack was not quite as good a student as Sally but he nonetheless did very well. He maintained a *B*+ average while starring on the football team. He was also a prince charming at the senior prom—the rough-and-tumble all-American boy in our family.

In a way, Jack was also a "first born"—he was first-born *male* in the Leman family. This often happens with the middle born, and we'll be talking more about that in chapter 2.

The middle born is the mediator and negotiator who avoids conflict. Paradoxically, the middle born is independent and has extreme loyalty to his peer group. He is a maverick with many friends. He usually leaves home first or finds his real companionship outside the home because he feels sort of left out of things in his own family.

My brother fits some of the above characteristics, but not all. He has turned out to be an extremely conscientious, well-organized, serious and scholarly Ph.D. in clinical psychology, with his own private practice. All these are traits of the first born and as I have pointed out, Jack was the first-born male in the Leman family.

And then there was Kevin. I came along five years after Jack, which in some cases might have made me what psychologists call a "quasi-only child."[3] Often, when the last child in the family comes along a good five or more years after the others, he starts a whole new birth order level. A child that much younger than his brothers or sisters is often left to himself and therefore knows something of being the "lonely only."

The only-child syndrome usually includes being treated like a little adult by your parents, who expect a lot from you. My older brother took all that pressure off me because of the expectations my parents placed directly on him. His official name was John E. Leman, JUNIOR. He was to be the medical doctor my father had always wanted to be but couldn't because he was very poor and only finished eighth grade. Dad projected onto Jack his own dreams of a fine profession and his own fears of "not being somebody." First borns and only children often become doctors, but my family never even considered any kind of career like that for me. When I was eleven days old I was nicknamed "Little Cub" and it stuck. Instead of being ignored and left to myself, I became the family mascot, who was always getting into something.

In fact, I learned very early that I had two "superstars" ahead of me and there really wasn't a whole lot I could do by way of the achievement trail to gain attention. My only real accomplishment while going through high school was playing on the baseball team (that is, when I was eligible—usually the first six weeks of the spring semester before grades came out). Jack never bothered with baseball. He chose football, which in most high schools is the major sport. In western New York, where we grew up, baseball is for the hardy types who are willing to put up with freezing to death before very small crowds in unpredictable spring weather.

But Little Cub wasn't going to be left out. He became manipulative, charming, a show-off, precocious, and engaging. At age eight, while trying to lead a cheer for my sister's high school team, I found my "true calling" in life. I learned that entertainers get attention. So, entertain I did, especially for my classmates all through grade school. I became something of a cross between the school terror and the school comedian. I had incredible skill at driving teachers a

22

little crazy, but more about all that in chapter 7, which will cover the youngest child in the family.

It All Comes Back to That Family Tree

I have no way of knowing what kind of family you grew up in, but it's my guess you could come up with a cast of characters similar to the Leman kids: the good students, the athletes, the performers, the attention getters, and the ones who are hard to pigeonhole. After about two decades of psychological study and practice, I am sure of only a few things:

1. *The most intimate relationships we ever have in life are with our families*—the one we grew up in and the one we make for ourselves through marriage.

2. *For a young child growing up, there is no greater influence than his or her family.* (Yes, I know about all the time they spend in school, Little League, Brownies; it's really a drop in the bucket compared to what goes on at home.)

3. *The relationship between parents and children is fluid, dynamic, and all-important.* Every time another child is born, *the entire family environment changes.* How parents interact with each child as it enters the family's circle determines in great part that child's final destiny.

I'm not sure if that last remark sounds profound or just a bit pontifical. All I know is that my father never had the opportunity to go beyond eighth grade, something he always regretted. He wanted very much for at least one of his sons to be a medical doctor. I don't think he was partial to doctors because of any visions of saving the world from disease and death. He just knew that doctors were well educated and well paid. Education became a major value that he communicated to all of his children—even bear cub Kevin, who didn't show as much promise as the older children.

Did this sink in? Well, the results tell their own story. First-born sister Sally got all *A*s all her life, right up through a master's program, which she uses in her preschool director work.

Brother Jack is a clinical psychologist, and somehow bear cub Kevin wound up a psychologist, too. Sally and Jack were no great surprise. They "had it right from the start." But how did Kevin, the "clown prince," get a doctor's degree? One answer is, "With a great deal of difficulty!" I'll tell you more about it in chapter 7, but for now let us leave it in the minor-miracle category. My high school teachers might even label it a *major* miracle.

4. *We don't spend enough time being aware of just how our branch fits on the family tree.* First born or lonely only, middle child or "baby"—all of us sprout in our own unique direction and make our own unique contributions. I believe that

reading this book will not only be enjoyable but very helpful as well. I see it happen every day. As people understand birth order, they improve relationships where it counts—with friends, on the job, and most important, at home with the people who are nearest, but not always dearest.

Of course, I realize you may still be a tiny bit skeptical. You may be like the guy who comes up to me and says, "Wait a minute, Leman. I heard a birth order talk [or read a birth order article] once. Those descriptions didn't fit my family at all. Furthermore, I'm a first born and it never did me any good. I never got any advantages."

And I just smile and nod and say, "Yes, it's obvious you were first born in your family's zoo. Sit down, and let me explain how it works. . . ."

Chapter Two

You and the Family Zoo

Every now and then someone—usually a first born because they tend to be more analytical and critical—confronts me with loud protests about how the "typical" descriptions of first-born, middle-born, and last-born children don't fit his (or her) family at all (or so it seems to him). I always appreciate this kind of interaction, because it helps me give that person deeper insights into birth order.

So, let's set up a conversation of the kind I often have after a seminar or workshop, or which sometimes takes place with a client I have just started counseling. For this scenario let's have me talking to "First Born Frank":

FIRST BORN FRANK   Your birth order system doesn't fit my family at all —you say first borns are neat. Well, I'm a first born and I'm known for having the sloppiest desk in the office. In fact, the last time anyone saw the top of my desk was the

	day before I started working for the company. So, what do you say to that, Doctor?
DR. LEMAN	That's interesting. What do you do for a living?
FIRST BORN FRANK	I'm an electrical engineer.
DR. LEMAN	Sounds like a very structured area—lots of math and mental discipline?
FIRST BORN FRANK	True enough, but how do you account for the sloppy desk?
DR. LEMAN	Your desk is sloppy—okay, but can you find what you need on it?
FIRST BORN FRANK	Of course. I usually know what's in every pile.
DR. LEMAN	So, you have order within your disorder? You are in a very disciplined occupation—engineering. And while your desk is sloppy, you still feel you are organized. My guess is you are something of a perfectionist and perfectionists are known for having sloppy desks as a means

of covering their discouragement for not always having life go just the way they want it. [We'll be looking more closely at the "discouraged perfectionist" in chapters 4 and 5.] Another thing about perfectionists—when they find one thing that is wrong or imperfect they tend to generalize that one inconsistency and want to throw out the entire package. Maybe you're trying to throw out the birth order baby with the bathwater.

FIRST BORN FRANK Well, I believe in being consistent and doing things right—and besides, your description of the youngest child in our family doesn't fit my sister at all. You said the baby of the family is manipulative, charming, precocious, engaging—a real sales type. My baby sister owns and operates her own interior decorating shop. Her biggest strength is organization and a good business head. And she's rather quiet, leaving the selling to the assistants. Actually, the engaging-salesman description is a perfect picture of my brother, Bill. He went into computer software sales and did so well he now has his own company, a big house, nice car, etc. . . .

DR. LEMAN   Let me ask you, are you and your brother more alike or opposite?

FIRST BORN FRANK   Oh, we're more opposite. I had only one good friend in high school and he had about two dozen. I ran the mile, he played football. When we got out of school he went into sales and I went into engineering. I used to kid him in high school because he couldn't do elementary algebra. He still can't do elementary algebra, but he makes three

29

times the money I do. He's very good at basic math—like bank deposits.

DR. LEMAN Okay, let me comment on you and your brother. It's very common—almost inevitable—that the second born turns out different from the first born. Every branch on the family tree seems to go in its own direction. Being first born, you had your eyes on Mom and Dad. They were the only models you had. You were more like the little adult—perfectionistic, reliable, conscientious, good at math—wanting things to be right. Your little brother looked up and saw big brother firmly planted in his spot and decided to go another route. Math wasn't for him—he would rather rap with his buddies. You ran the mile, a loner's kind of sport. He played

	on the football team—where his friends were.
FIRST BORN FRANK	What about my baby sister, Nancy? How do you explain her?
DR. LEMAN	Okay, hold on to your hat. Nancy was born *third* in your family, but she was the *first-born female.* It's my guess that your brother Bill was more the baby of the family than Nancy was. You probably snowplowed the roads of life for him and he learned to depend on competent big brother—at least until he could go out and find his own friends. And, let me ask you, how many years between your brother Bill and baby sister Nancy?
FIRST BORN FRANK	Nancy is six years younger than Bill—and you're right—Mom made me baby-sit him quite a bit until he got into third grade. It was a drag—in fact, he was very good at pestering me and then

31

	screaming bloody murder if I clipped him one. Now that I think about it, he was a master at setting me up.
DR. LEMAN	That's not surprising. Now let's look at Nancy. She was born last but late. She was supposedly the baby of the family, but she was born so far from you and Bill that she probably grew up as an only child. And remember, she was the first-born girl—that's also important. You and Bill could easily have been more like uncles to her than brothers. Did either of you do a lot with Nancy?
FIRST BORN FRANK	Not really. We were both into our own thing. I was in junior high and Bill was into Little League—his own buddies.
DR. LEMAN	Then it's really not that surprising that Nancy developed traits of a first born—quiet, organized,

probably spent quite a bit of her time playing alone. . . .

FIRST BORN FRANK

I suppose she did. Well, you wiggled out of that one, too! At least I made you work for it. I like to grill you psychologists about your theories. It looks to me as if you can make birth order just about anything you want it to be.

DR. LEMAN

Not on your slide rule, Frank! But what our little chat does prove is that you are definitely a first born—very skeptical, analytical, organized, precise in your thinking. I'm glad you challenged me on the "typical" description of first, second, and last born. The truth is, those typical descriptions are only general statements. People can differ depending on when they were born, their sex, the family situation at the time—all these forces are at work. Psychological jargon for this is the "family constellation." I like to call it the Family Zoo—but whatever you call it, every family has its own mix.

Every Family Zoo Is Different

My chat with First-Born Frank was hypothetical, but still based on many such discussions I've had with people who have challenged me on birth order theory. The so-called inconsistencies that folks point out are only signposts pointing to the most entertaining and interesting part of birth order theory—what I like to call the Family Zoo. (You may prefer the more dignified term, "family constellation," but because I deal with many a desperate mother who has three or four little "munchkins" driving her crazy, it's easy to see why "zoo" comes to mind.)

Birth order isn't a simplistic 1-2-3 system that says all first borns are equally one way, all second children are another, and last-born kids are always just like this or that. There are tendencies and general characteristics that often apply, but the real point is that there are dynamic relationships existing between members of a family. They all live in the same den, so to speak, but they are distinctly different. How can two or three or more kids come from the same parents, live in the same house, and become so different? That's the real question, and birth order helps answer it, as long as you are aware of the variables affecting each family situation.

And what are these "variables"? I believe they include spacing (the number of years between children), the sex of each child, physical differences or disabilities, the birth order position of the parents, any blending of two or more families due to death or divorce, and finally, the relationship between the parents. Let's look at these one at a time and diagram some possible combinations that can radically affect the constellation, or grouping, of each family.

Spacing Can Create More Than One "Family"

An obvious—and crucial—birth order variable in any family is the spacing of children. Just when does each child arrive? Many people try to have their children two years apart (actually three is "ideal"), but it seldom works out that way. What we often find are gaps in the spacing of the children, which can sometimes create what amounts to another "family." Whenever there is a gap of five or more years, it often means that a "second family" has begun. The diagram of Family A shows how this can happen:

FAMILY A
    Male — 14
    Female — 13

    Male — 6
    Female — 5

The dotted line depicts the obvious split in this kind of birth order ranking. The gap of seven years between the second- and third-born children creates a situation that could easily result in the third-born boy developing first-born tendencies. This doesn't mean he would have no characteristics of a middle child (in a family of four children, numbers two and three rank as "middle" children). He could still become a negotiator; he could still have a lot of friends. But he also might be quite "adult"—conscientious, exacting—because he had so many older models. Not only would his parents model adult characteristics for him, but so would his much bigger brother and sister.

One other thing about Family A: with the "older" family (the fourteen- and thirteen-year-olds), you could have two basic combinations. You might wind up with a first-born male and a first-born female, or a first-born male and a "baby princess." A lot would depend upon the family values.

For example, in a very traditional home the oldest male usually gets the "manly" chores such as cutting the lawn, digging weeds, hauling trash, and helping Dad. His younger sister would be assigned the "mother's helper" kind of jobs: ironing, housecleaning, doing the dishes, and so on. In this family the younger sister is more likely to become "baby princess" rather than "first-born female." She will be taught to be very feminine, while the macho activities are left to her brother.

Then, seven years later, in the traditional family we might do it all over again with another "first born" boy and a younger sister who turns out to be another "baby princess." But let's suppose we change the values in Family A. Let's suppose the parents are a bit more "liberated" and decide all their kids will share equally in the chores. The boys get to do the dishes and other housework. The girls get a shot at running a lawn mower. Now we have a situation that could produce a first-born boy and first-born girl, followed seven or eight years later by another first-born boy and first-born girl. There would never be a bona fide "baby princess" because family values wouldn't give much opportunity for her to develop.

The Sex of Each Child Can Cause Pressure Points

We've already mentioned one way sex can affect birth order by showing how a third-born child can become the "first born girl." But it really gets interesting when you end up with something like four boys and one girl. You don't have to be a certified psychologist to figure out there is something special about one member of that family! And, depending upon where the girl is placed in the family constellation, the effect on at least one of her brothers can be anything from substantial to awesome. For example, let's take a look at Family B:

FAMILY B
Male   —   16
Male   —   14
Male   —   12
Female —   11
Male   —   9

With this kind of mix, which child do you think is in the least preferable position? If you guessed the third-born male (the twelve-year-old) you hit it on the nose. But why him? Because Mom has already been down to the hospital three times and brought home a boy every time, so it's getting to be old hat. The parents have been pulling for a girl and now here she is, fourth born, a very special baby princess, and only fifteen to eighteen months behind our third-born male. He is bound to hear her footsteps, even before she can walk!

Just for a little more intrigue, *who else* might feel the pressure from baby princess? Yep, irony of ironies, it will be the last-born male. He is the "baby of the family" by birth order, but big sister beat him to the punch. Chances are, after three boys in a row, she is apple of Daddy's (and Mommy's) eye. Now, two years later, here comes little Festus, the caboose. He doesn't get the usual attention given the last born because Mom and Dad already have three boys but only one girl, who is almost certain to be given special treatment.

Chances are it will be tough for Festus to get his share of the attention. You can make a pretty good guess that our little nine-year-old is an attention getter of one kind or another. He has probably learned to live by his wits and, if so blessed, by his nimble feet. Three older brothers are always ready to try to lose him in the woods or pound him black and blue (particularly if he bugs them to get attention).

With all that competition ahead of him, little Festus could easily decide that he will be best at being worst, which is exactly what I did as youngest child with two superstars ahead of me. Festus could be a mischief, even a delinquent; or he could decide to play helpless wonder of the world. At school he might become an academic zero or even "behaviorally disturbed." On a milder note, he might become a nonreader who needs constant drill by Mom or Dad.

Who is the boy in the family in the best spot? A good bet, of course, is the first-born male, who will be likely to excel at school. He will also be likely to engage in plenty of rivalry with his younger brother because any time the second born is of the same sex as the first born, there is bound to be more friction. If older brother is a scholar, second born is likely to be an athlete, or he may prefer the school band and leave the athletics for the third-born boy. If the third-born does become an athlete, it could be his salvation because it will help him to work out the frustration caused by having to compete with baby princess.

That's just one example of how the sex of the child can affect the family. The rule of thumb is this: When sex differences create someone "special" it can put pressure on the children immediately above or below that special person.

In This Corner, Burly the Bigger!

Another variable that can turn the birth order factor upside down or at least tilt it a bit sideways is marked difference in physical makeup or ability. Suppose we have little Chester, age ten.

He is oldest, but he is still called "little." Why? Because he has a brother only one year younger named Burly, who is four inches taller and who outweighs him by twenty-five pounds.

In this situation, a two-child family, both males, natural rivalry intense, Chester had better be extra quick or extra smart or he's in trouble!

Let's take another all-too-frequent example. Samantha, twelve, the first-born girl, is extremely pretty and Abigail, ten, second-born (and last) child is absolutely plain. As Dr. James Dobson has so accurately pointed out in *Hide or Seek,* Abigail is a classic candidate for a poor self-image. Beauty is, indeed, the gold coin of human worth.[1] It is sad but true that adults will respond better to cute little Sammy than they will to plain little Abby. If Abby can't find some kind of "secret weapon," such as being the athlete or maybe the family scholar, she's in for a long and dreary career as "Sammy's homely little sister."

Now let's expand the number in the family to four and have one suffer from a serious disease. Family C gives us one such combination:

FAMILY C
    Male — 14
    Male — 12
    Female — 10 (cerebral palsy victim)
    Female — 8

Here we have a family with a special person indeed. The first thing we can pretty well guess is that the eight-year-old girl isn't going to be the baby in the family—she will take the role of first-born female. This is called a "role reversal" —where two children do something of a flip-flop. The first-born girl, victim of a serious physical disability, becomes the "baby" and youngest sister takes on the role of first-born girl (as well as becoming something of a "middle" child in the family).

And what about the two older brothers? Chances are they're going to grow up to be two caring males who are sensitive toward women. They will spend an awful lot of time serving and caring for their handicapped sister. They probably won't always be crazy about doing it, but the realities of life will mold them into more sensitive men than they would have been had their sister been physically whole.

Let me give you one more example of a physical difference that isn't as visible, but it's all too real. Our constellation in Family D reads:

FAMILY D
    Female — 10

Here we have the only child—often called "the lonely only." In this case, she may or may not be lonely, but she is definitely ruling the roost. Since infancy she has been in charge and it gets worse every year. Now—at age ten—she doesn't simply boss Mom and Dad, she also rips them off! If they won't give her what she wants, she steals it.

I have counseled cases like this and it doesn't take long to get some vital information (and explanations). Before little Helen was born, Mom had two miscarriages. This is a very big clue as to why Helen has turned out to be an unholy terror. After two miscarriages, a woman can be shopping in the supermarket and see a mother with her new baby. The odds are excellent she will start to bawl even though the onions are sixty feet away. After two heartbreaking miscarriages, Mom wanted to have Helen so badly that when she finally arrived it was more than significant, and it was even more than special.

We parents can do a lot of wrong things in the name of love and in Helen's case Mom (and Dad) did only one, but they did it up big. It's called *overindulgence.* The "physical difference" in this case was the two dead siblings, lost through miscarriage, and a very alive little Helen. Mom and Dad didn't just spoil Helen, they made every day a Disneyland. By age ten she was taking them for every ride in the book! It takes a lot of patience and determination to turn this kind of family around. To be candid, I am glad if I bat .500.

When the Parents Were Born Counts, Too

So far we have only talked about birth order variables among children. How about parents? The order in which parents are born can also be a critical influence on the family constellation. How does a mom's or dad's order of birth affect their children? One typical force at work is the tendency for a parent to overidentify with the child in the same birth order position he or she shares.

I can recall a child psychology class I taught as an adjunct professor at the University of Arizona. One morning we did a "family constellation demonstration" in front of two hundred students, most of whom were employed as teachers or counselors. I brought in a mother, a father, and three children and had an interesting time interacting with all of them in front of the class.

Afterward, when the family had gone, I asked the group for some feedback. Because most of them were not neophytes, but practicing professionals, I was curious about their reactions. There were different observations, but most of them agreed on one thing: "It seems as if you paid an awful lot of attention to the baby of the family—the four-year-old girl."

Without thinking too much about it, I said, "Yeah, wasn't she cute?"

But then it hit me. Of course I thought the baby was cute! I'm the baby in my family, too! I made a career of being cute and funny all through school and beyond.

And come to think about it, when I interact with my own three children, whose antics do I enjoy the most? Kevin II, our baby, of course! When Holly, our oldest, now fourteen, or Krissy, our middle child, now thirteen, comes and complains about nine-year-old Kevey and his pestering ways, I say, "Well, honey, let's remember he's the baby of the family . . . little baby brothers do that kind of thing to sisters."

On the other hand, I tend to be a bit more stern if the tattler's shoe is on Kevin's foot and he complains about Holly, our oldest. We tend to expect more of the older kids, particularly our first born, right? But would I be as strict with Holly if I were the first born in my family? I'm not so sure. I know I'm not alone in overidentifying with the child closest to me in birth order. I see it in too many families I counsel.

Let's use the diagram of Family E to look at an example where both parents are first born:

FAMILY E

Husband — first-born dentist	Wife — first-born PTA president

Female — 16
Female — 14
Female — 12

Who is in best position in this family? In this case, the parents may "overidentify" with the sixteen-year-old first born, but not in an indulging way. The oldest girl is likely to get pummeled by the perfectionistic standards of her two first-born parents. *Their* way of overidentifying will center in pressuring oldest daughter to do her best.

Actually, the child in the best position in the family could be number two, because big sister has run interference for her to some extent and absorbed a lot of the perfectionistic energy that two first-born parents would likely pour into their first child.

What about the third born—the "baby"—of this particular family constellation? Remember, parents tend to identify with the child nearest them in birth order. So, chances are, the first-born dentist and the first-born PTA president won't be too enamored with any of third born's precocious or manipulative ways.

In this family—in *any* family, for that matter—a lot depends on parenting style. If Mom and Dad are two authoritarians, that is, if they come down too hard and too unreasonably, they can turn the oldest girl into a rebel. She could be a good candidate to foul up in school, maybe on purpose, just to foil the plans of her "perfect parents."

On the other hand, if these parents have read some good advice (for example, my book *Mak-*

ing Children Mind Without Losing Yours), they may understand the difference between hard-nosed authoritarianism and a balanced authoritative style that makes demands but is fair and reasonable.

With a reasonable, authoritative style, these first-born parents could push their sixteen-year-old to graduate from high school and go on to be an aeronautical engineer. Or who knows? She could wind up an astronaut or maybe an airline pilot. Not long ago, a Frontier Airlines flight was piloted and copiloted by two women —the first event of its kind for a major airline.

What Happens When Two Families Blend?

The answer is plenty! As a therapist who does his share of counseling with stepfamilies, I am tempted to advise, "Love is seldom lovelier the second time around." I'm not trying to be cynical or negative, but the statistics are overwhelming. Handling first borns, middle borns, and last borns in one family is challenging enough, but when you bring two families together, in "Brady Bunch" fashion, it can really get complicated.

I might add that the writers of "The Brady Bunch" must have worked wearing rose-colored glasses. The "problems" or "crises" faced by the

Brady family somehow always seemed to be neatly solved in thirty minutes and everyone lived happily ever after. In real blended families, it is seldom that simple, for several reasons.

If You're About to Get Stepped On

When I learn that someone with children is considering remarriage with someone else with children, I try to tell them, "You can get stepped on in a stepfamily." The odds against second marriages are long at best. It's tough enough if only one of the partners brings children to the new marriage, but add the complications of two sets of children living with the new mom and dad under the same roof and it can be tough—*very* tough. While a lot of people know all about these odds, it doesn't seem to deter them. It is naive to expect "instant love" among all members of a stepfamily, but people often remarry, believing "It will be different with us." Stepparents acquire instant children, all right, but instead of experiencing instant love, they usually get instant problems. A stepfather or stepmother must realize that his new stepchildren have had special relationships in their other family for years. In comparison, the relationship a remarried partner has with his or her spouse is usually two years old at most, usually less. It is totally unreasonable to think that a two-year-old relationship is going to outweigh parent-child relationships that have existed for ten or twelve years, or whatever age the children may be. To paraphrase the old saying, blood in biological families is thicker than the punch served at the remarriage ceremony.

A key factor in how successfully a stepfamily can build loving relationships is the age of the children at the time of the new marriage. If the children are young, for example, stepsisters age one and three joined with stepbrothers age two and four, the odds are much better. Their personalities are still being formed and time is on the parents' side.

But suppose the children are older—for example, a ten-year-old girl is joined to a stepsister, thirteen, and a stepbrother, fifteen. Now we are talking about personalities and relationships that are well formed. To build new relationships among everyone concerned in the family will take time, patience—and maybe some luck.

Making the Pieces Fit

To illustrate the difficulties facing the blended family, let's take a quick look at what happens to the birth order factor when Mom brings her kids to a second marriage and Dad brings his. They all hope for instant love and harmony when what they can easily have, as the diagram shows, is instant war!

FAMILY F

Father's Children	Mother's Children
Male — 12	Male — 13
Male — 11	Male — 10
Female — 9	Female — 8

In this constellation there almost has to be thunder and lightning. Each set of first, second, and third borns are paired off in natural competition for their piece of the pie. If I see people considering this kind of marriage, my first suggestion is "Don't do it!" It is almost a no-win situation.

If this kind of combination comes to me as an already blended family, I am tempted to say a bit facetiously, "Your only hope is to sell the children. You could get a good price for them on the coast!"

Of course, we don't really suggest selling the kids, but it's tempting. In many stepfamily situations the children are the enemy. It is quite normal for them to wish (and work) for the new marriage to fail. Why? Because they are still loyal to the missing natural parent or parents. They can't accept Mom or Dad living with somebody else.

Is every blended family in as much potential trouble as Family F? Let's look at two more examples and you tell me who might have more problems.

FAMILY G

Father's Children	Mother's Children
Male — 16	Female — 11
Male — 14	Female — 9
	Male — 4

FAMILY H

Father's Children	Mother's Children
Female — 14	Female — 13
Female — 10	Male — 10
	Female — 8

Which couple would you bet on to make their blended family work? The odds aren't very good for blended Family H. They have the same "natural" competition problem as did Family F: two first-born females, fourteen and thirteen, vying for top spot, two ten-year-old second borns feeling more squeezed than ever as they try to find room in the middle, and on Mom's side, eight-year-old baby princess wondering how she can charm, tease, or even cheat her way into the spotlight.

Your best bet is really blended Family G. No one is coming in to seriously challenge the sixteen-year-old male's first-born turf. He and his second-born brother have had an understanding for fourteen years. Over on Mom's side, the four-year-old male is just a "little twerp"—in fact, the older boys may decide to make him a bear cub mascot, if he plays his cards right.

As for the girls, at ages nine and eleven, they won't prove any problem for the sixteen-year-old. They'll be happy to play their video games or watch TV.

If there's going to be any friction in blended Family G, it can start with the fourteen-year-old male on Dad's side and any one of the three kids from Mom's side. For fourteen years he has been baby in his family and now all of a sudden, three new "babies" have all slipped in beneath him to compete for his special spot. The most likely problem could be the eleven-year-old first born from Mom's side. For eleven years, she has been ruling the roost in her own family. Now, forced into an artificial role as a "middle child," she may not want to take on the sixteen-year-old stepbrother, but depending upon how feisty she is, she may decide the fourteen-year-old is fair game.

All in all, though, blended Family G has a good shot at making it, as long as Mom and Dad can get along. In fact, in any family—and especially the stepfamily—the relationship between the parents is the most vital variable influencing everything. The secret of success for any marriage is to put yourselves, not your children, first. We will be taking a closer look at all this in chapters 8 and 9, which deal with birth order and marriage.

Twins Stand Out in Any Birth Order

Whether fraternal (born from separate eggs and with few resemblances) or identical (born from one egg and look-alikes), twins are a very special event. When talking to twins a key question is, "Who was born first?" One usually is quick to let you know, "I'm older," even if it's by as little as one minute!

Twins are often an interesting mix of competitor and companion. The "first born" often takes the assertive role of leader while the "second born" follows along. I say often, but not always. Some twinships turn into real rivalries, especially when the children are the same sex.[2]

When you come to the family constellation, twins are bound to cause pressure—especially on any children born after them. For example, let's look at the diagram of Family I:

FAMILY I
    Female — 12
    Male — 10
    Males — 7 and 7
    Female — 3

Here we have twin boys, with a first-born sister and first-born brother above them. The older children will probably be able to handle the special attention paid to the twins, but the last-born child is going to have problems, even though she is a baby princess. She will, however, have a better chance than a last-born boy would.

Obviously, the best time for twins to be born would be last, and this is often the case because women in their forties are much more likely to have twins than women in their twenties.[3]

Birth Order Helps Makes Us Unique

This short course in the workings of the Family Zoo (constellation) should help illustrate how birth order works to make us unique individuals. When we mix our order of birth with the variable forces we've looked at in this chapter, we get some good clues as to why we are the way we are. Of course, there is no way to always accurately predict how any one person may turn out. We are all too different and complex—too unique. Only God, who knows us even while we're in our mother's womb,[4] has the whole picture. What we can be sure of are the following:

1. *Living in a family is a unique and distinctive experience.* In every family is a set of intimate relationships you can find nowhere else on earth.[5]

Those relationships are created in great part by your order of birth.

2. *A person's family exerts more influence on him or her than any other organization, institution, or experience.* Schools, churches, teens, clubs, colleges, and jobs all come later in life, after those early years of imprinting that mold so much of one's basic personality. And, later in life, family influence persists, even across the miles when children grow up and move away.[6]

3. *In any family, a person's order of birth has a lifelong effect on who and what that person turns out to be.* Are you an only or first born? You are a different person than you would have been had you been born later. Are you the baby in the family? Things would be different, and so would you, had you been born first. Are you the "squeezed" middle child? You can look up or possibly down and think about how it might have been had you been born earlier or later.

4. *No matter what spot we occupy in the family, there are many forces that can intervene and turn things around for us.* I realize that I made the blended family examples sound "pretty hopeless." Friction, trouble, frustration, and even war all seemed inevitable. But with proper intervention by those in helping professions, relationships can be vastly improved.

And there is, of course, the most powerful intervention of all—finding a real relationship to God and/or practicing your faith with wholehearted commitment. As a Bible-believing Christian, I do not push my faith on others, but I do share my beliefs when the opportunity presents itself. I have seen incredible turn-arounds in the most hopeless kinds of situations, simply because people circumvented or rose above their problems and weaknesses with the power that comes through faith.[7]

Now that we've gotten our feet wet in birth order thinking, let's go into a little deeper water and take a closer look at each of the three major birth orders. In honor of First Born Fred, we'll start with him.

Part Two

The Special Burden of All First Borns

It is always a bit rash to saddle any birth order with a blanket label, but first borns, and their close cousins, the only children, have one. It's *perfectionism,* which in extreme cases can result in slow suicide. First borns and only children get a lot of attention, a lot of glory—and a lot of pressure. In the next three chapters we'll take a look at . . .

- the game first borns almost always win
- why some first borns attract the "great white sharks" of life
- why other first borns *hunt* the great white sharks of life
- why history's first first born committed homicide
- why first borns get the most discipline
- why first borns have to grow up fast

- why only children are often lonely and unpopular
- why only children seldom feel "good enough"
- the perfectionist wife who ran herself ragged
- why slobs can still be perfectionists
- tips to help perfectionists live more happily with themselves and others

Chapter Three

First Born: First Come, First Served

When I'm on the road doing family and parenting seminars, I have a favorite little "lab exercise" that I use to help people get in touch with their birth order characteristics—and at the same time it helps me get a better idea of who I am working with and how I can help them the most.

The exercise works like this:

I ask the seminar participants to divide into several groups with only children in one corner, first borns in a second, middle borns in a third, and last borns (the family babies) over in the far corner where they won't bother anyone but themselves. I don't give the groups any instructions at this point, except to say, "Just chat a bit, but remain in your circle."

Next I move around the room as unobtrusively as possible and slip a piece of paper into the center of each circle and leave it lying facedown on the floor. I still give no instructions —at least out loud. Each piece of paper has the same instructions, turned facedown, which read: "Congratulations! you are the leader of this group. Please introduce yourself to the others in your group, and then have each person do the same. As you talk together, make a list of personality characteristics that you all seem to share. Be prepared to report back to the rest of the seminar with your 'composite picture' of yourselves. Please start work immediately."

What usually happens? First, all the groups keep waiting for me to give some kind of verbal instruction. When none is forthcoming, it is interesting to watch "birth order nature" take its course. Who picks up the piece of paper first? Almost invariably someone in the only-born or first-born group picks up the paper and reads the instructions. Not long after, the middle borns follow suit. Soon, three groups in the room are busy with their assignments.

And the fourth group? Well, the last borns are usually still milling around, while their piece of paper remains on the floor, unread.

I wait a little longer and finally make one announcement: "You have only a few more minutes to finish your assignment. Be ready to report to the rest of the seminar at that time!"

The only borns and the first borns look up like startled deer and then redouble their efforts to finish their assigned tasks. The middles don't look quite as impressed, but they do try to press on toward the finish. As for the last borns, they're having such a good time they usually don't even hear what I said.

During one seminar I conducted, the babies all milled around in the far corner, their circle looking more like a figure eight than anything else, as they had a high old time. One man wound up standing on the piece of paper that had originally been placed in the center of his circle!

I don't tell the story to make fun of the babies in the family. I'm a baby in my family myself and I'm sure that, placed in the same situation, I'd be the guy standing on the piece of paper! But in the almost two hundred times I've conducted this exercise, I can remember only one or two cases where the first people to pick up the piece of paper and start "obeying instructions" did *not* come from the first- or only-born circles. If you will recall the little quiz we took in chapter 1, the "typical characteristics" of first- or only-born people include: perfectionistic, reliable, conscientious, list makers, well organized, critical, serious, scholarly.

To that list you could add: goal oriented, achiever, self-sacrificing, people pleaser, conservative, supporter of law and order, believer in authority and ritual, legalistic, loyal, self-reliant.

In most books that talk about birth order, the first borns usually get more than their share of the coverage. This is not too surprising because first borns usually get more ink in the write-ups of life. They are often the achievers, the ones who are driven toward success and stardom in their given fields.

You can't ignore the first borns. If you aren't one, you have to deal with them somewhere along the line. In some cases it can mean friction, even war. Maybe your older first-born brother or sister wound up as your baby-sitter, something that didn't set that well with either of you. On the other hand, some first borns become champion, even second parent, to their younger brothers or sisters. That's what happened with me and my first-born sister, Sally.

What Makes the First Born Run?

There are at least two good reasons first borns usually come in such downright-upright (and sometimes a little uptight) packages. Those two reasons are Mom and Dad. Brand-new parents tend to be a paradox when it comes to their first-born child. One side of them is overprotective, anxious, tentative, and inconsistent. The other side can be strict in discipline, demanding, always pushing and encouraging more and better performance.

The simple truth is, the first born is something of a guinea pig as Mom and Dad try to learn the fine art of parenting. After all, they have never done any of this before. *Everything* about the first-born child is a big deal and it starts well before little Festus or Mildred arrives. While Mom is pregnant, the very air is charged with expectancy in more ways than one. Imagine (or remember for yourself) the grand anticipation of the young parents as they celebrate with baby showers, picking out names, choosing wallpaper for the nursery, buying baby clothes and toys. (If the parents are first borns or only borns themselves, add to that list piggy banks, insurance policies, and choice of college or university.)

There is little doubt that the family sort of overdoes things with the first born. If grandparents are nearby they always add to the fun of recording every cry, look, whim, or move on video, movie camera, or at least Grandma's old faithful Instamatic. It's not surprising that research indicates first borns walk and talk earlier than later borns. With all the coaching, prodding, and encouragement they get, they probably do it in self-defense!

Another thing about your typical first borns is that they are often serious. Life is real and life is earnest for the first-born individual. He or she isn't much for surprises. First borns prefer to know what's happening and when. They thrive on being in control, on time, and organized.

First borns automatically fit into the category labeled "advanced." It isn't their idea, but with only adults for models they naturally take on more adult characteristics. First-born people usually grow up to be conservative. With all that adult input and pressure to perform, they become the family standard-bearers. First-born children are "little adults" who often go on to become the leaders and achievers in life.

Are All First Borns Alike?

I've been painting first-born people with some pretty broad brush strokes: organized, overparented, overprotected, pressured to perform, achievers, conservative, and wanting control. But of course it is never that simple. With first borns in particular, you can have two basic types: compliant and wanting to please, or strong willed and aggressive.

Your compliant first born is the "model child" who grows up to be a pleaser of others. Compliant first borns are the reliable, conscientious wonders of the world. When they're asked to do something, they say, "Yes, Mom . . . Yes, Dad . . . Yes, sir . . . No, sir, I'll be glad to do it." Who doesn't want a few children or employees like that around? They tend to be good students and good workers. They have a very strong *need for approval*. They want Mom and Dad to approve; they want the boss to approve; they want their spouse to approve.

My wife, Sande, is a perfect example of a compliant first born. Not too far from our home in Tucson, Arizona, there is a five-star restaurant

that would be considered among the finest anywhere. Every now and then, on very special occasions, Sande and I go there for dinner. During
one of our visits, we had both ordered our meal
and it came, served in the usual impeccable and
precise manner. As I ate, I glanced over at Sande
and noticed that she was simply picking around
the edges of her poached salmon.

"How's your dinner?" I asked. "Is everything
okay?"

"Oh . . . yes. Everything's just great. Isn't
this one of the nicest restaurants you could ever
ask for?"

But as I continued eating I noticed that Sande
continued picking and not really getting into
that poached salmon. Finally, I zeroed in on the
problem: "Tell me, is your salmon really done
to your liking? You just aren't eating it."

"Well . . . it really is not quite cooked in the
middle."

It turned out the "poached" salmon was so
raw it could have passed for sushi. Being a last-
born child of the family and not at all compliant,
I quickly summoned the waiter and made him
aware of the problem. The waiter, not to mention the maître d' and chef, was horrified! He
rushed the salmon out to the kitchen and a short
while later an entirely new serving of the salmon
appeared, cooked to perfection. Not only that,
but a little later the chef sent out a special
"peace offering" in the form of a gigantic Baked

Alaska dessert, "compliments of the house with apologies to madam for the inconvenience."[1]

I tell the story not to give you tips on how to be assertive with waiters or get special desserts free of charge, but to illustrate Sande's compliant, "I'd rather not complain about it but just bear with it" nature. Sande is a pleaser, a nurturer, and a care giver, all classic characteristics of the compliant first born.

Compliant first borns can often attract the "great white sharks" of life who like to take a chunk out of them now and then. I often counsel this kind of person. The classic scenario finds a man who has been working in middle management for several years at a big corporation. His superintendent or manager—perhaps it's a vice-president—has a way of piling on the work. He keeps coming by and dropping little projects on this guy's desk. He also has a way of making it very clear that his evaluation will be coming up in May.

This first born who wants to please him has several things working against him. One is that he has a wife and four kids at home who need feeding and a few other things. But the even bigger psychological hammer that keeps pounding him is that ever since childhood he's felt that he was the responsible one who had to get everything done. He's the one who had to take out the garbage, cut the grass, etc., because his brothers and sisters were too little or perhaps undependable. Parents have a way of depending on their first-born child. I call it the "let George the first born do it" syndrome.

Team this kind of compliant first born up with a selfish, narcissistic boss or spouse and you have the makings for what could turn out to be trouble down the line. Compliant first borns are well known for "taking it" and being walked on by a world that loves to take advantage of them, but they also are known for nursing their resentments quietly and then eventually venting with one grand explosion.

While compliant first borns have a strong need to be conscientious, care giving, and servants, there is another brand of first born who is more assertive and strong willed. In some cases these power-driven first borns can acquire some badgerlike qualities. They develop traits that make them high achievers and hard drivers. They have high expectations and a strong need to be "kingpin."

One example of the hard-driving badger is the classic first-born executive who goes around uptight and immersed in his work for fifty weeks a year. Then he gets a two-week vacation and becomes a different person. Wives have told me, "When we go on vacation, Harry is just great. He relaxes and lets his hair down. He's almost normal with the kids and with me. But about *two* days before vacation is over, you can see him change. The look comes back on his face. And on the way home, his old hard-driving personality is already back."

The person with the hard-driving personality is often quite proud of the way he gets things done, but he pays the price. If his body doesn't break down, relationships with his family or friends usually do. History is full of hard-driving first borns who ended tragically. In the Old Testament it started early when Adam and Eve's first-born child, Cain, thought his sacrifice was every bit as good or better than his brother Abel's. When God didn't accept Cain's "fruit of the ground" he responded by making his brother, Abel, the first homicide victim in recorded history.[2]

On a much milder, but still very real note, Sande and I know a little about strong-willed first borns because we have one. Her name is Holly and as this book is being developed she is in the latter stages of that interesting period called preadolescence. That means she is twelve going on seventeen. Holly is bright, meticulous, and stubborn. One example of how precise and insistent Holly can be is that you don't answer a question like "What time are we going to leave?" by telling her, "Oh, pretty soon," or "Oh, somewhere around nine o'clock." To Holly it's far better to say, "We'll drive out of the parking lot at precisely 9:07 P.M.!"

Being First Has Its "Perks"

As I mentioned earlier, the first borns of this world undoubtedly get more attention and notoriety than anyone else. *Anything* first-born children do is a big deal as far as Mom and Dad and other members of the family are concerned. They get all kinds of attention and encouragement to achieve. That was certainly the case with my oldest sister, Sally, as well as my older brother, Jack, who was the first-born male in the family. Sally and Jack were supposed to carry the family banner to greater heights, and in many ways, they did.

A common characteristic of a first-born person is his confidence in being taken seriously by those around him. This comes from his childhood, when adults took him seriously and he knew it. It's no wonder that first borns often go on to positions of leadership or high achievement. Fifty-two percent of United States presidents were first borns (only four have been the babies in their families). First borns are over-represented among *Who's Who in America* and *American Men and Women of Science,* as well as among Rhodes scholars and university professors.[3]

First borns are known for strong powers of concentration, tolerance and patience, and being organized and conscientious. All of these traits give them a distinct advantage in many professions. For example, if you were manager of a bank and were hiring more tellers, whom would you choose? I have asked this question at seminars and some people say they would prefer the last-born children—the babies of families—because their friendliness and outgoing charm would be great assets in working with the public. But I always have to disagree and opt to hire first borns instead. True, it helps to be friendly when you are working with the public but it would be all too typical for a last-born bank teller to say something like this: "Margery, could you come here, please? Would you relieve me—I've got to have a Coke and there are still fourteen people in my line."

And there would also be that little problem of losing things—a natural trait with the babies of the family: "Let's see, I know that fifty thousand dollars is around here someplace. . . ."

Now remember, if you are a baby of the family and happen to be a bank teller or in some similar occupation, I am *not* saying you automatically are the type who might be less conscientious when the work load gets heavy or one who might carelessly lose large sums of money. The law of averages says, however, that the first born is a much better bet to be careful, conscientious, and "perfectionistic"—all important traits for someone entrusted with a lot of responsibility. First borns don't like to make mistakes. They are careful and calculating and they are sticklers for rules and regulations. All of these characteristics are useful for getting along well when working in fussy, precise places, like banks.

And Being First Born Has Its Problems

The old saying is so true, it's frightening: "Your strength is usually your weakness." The principle particularly applies to first borns. All of the attention, the oohing and aahing, the spotlight, and the responsibility add up to one thing—PRESSURE!

A lot of the pressure on the oldest child comes in the form of discipline and, in too many cases, punishment. Ask any first born and he or she will admit (maybe complain) about getting the heavy end of the hickory stick. First borns will tell you that they had to toe the mark while their younger brothers or sisters had it easier, at least to some degree. The simple truth is, as each child is added to the typical family, the rules and regulations are relaxed a little more. Has this happened in the Leman household, where Reality Discipline is supposed to be practiced unerringly by the expert psychologist and his loving wife? Holly, our eldest, and even Krissy, our second born, will probably tell you, "We have to toe the line, and Kevey gets away with murder!"

In defense of Sande and myself, we work extra hard at never treating all the children the same, but still try to be consistent when it comes to bedtime and other regulations. In other words, if Holly had to go to bed at eight o'clock when she was seven, so did Krissy, and so does Kevey. More on all this in the parenting section coming up in chapters 10 through 14.

Right along with getting the most discipline, the first born gets the most work. When something needs to be done in the family, whom do we call on? The first born is likely to draw the assignment, whether it is housework, an errand, or picking up dog flops. In fact, one of the chief complaints of most first-born adults is remembering being "left in charge" of younger brothers and sisters when they would have preferred to be off playing with their own friends. True, first borns might enjoy the baby-sitting role for a while, but it soon turns into a drag. In fact, it's not unusual for the older children to try and ditch younger ones who tag along. In the front of this book you may have noticed my special recognition of my brother, Jack, first-born male in our family, who often tried to lose his baby brother Kevin in the woods! A good rule of thumb is not to expect your older children to be baby-sitters for the young ones. But, of course, that is a rule that often gets broken, due to finances, unforeseen emergencies, or overloaded schedules.

For one reason or another we expect too much of first borns. We make them the pacesetters and standard-bearers of the family. They are often forced to follow in fathers' and mothers' footsteps as far as professions are concerned. The conflict between Dad, who wants his first-born son to take over the family business, and son, who wants to be a forest ranger, Peace Corps worker, or maybe even a missionary, is well known.

When the first born is a boy, there is a great deal of pressure on him to be "crown prince." With nothing but adult role models to go by—namely Mom and Dad—the prince is more like a little adult. And what is his first proving ground? The little red schoolhouse, of course. The record on first-born children is that they thrive in school. Getting good grades is something they can do easily to satisfy Mom's and Dad's expectations. And so, first borns usually do quite well in school. Of course, the motivation is there. Every little paper, every little drawing or piece of craft they bring home gets great reviews from Mom and Dad, not to mention Grandma and Grandpa. First borns often occupy center stage on refrigerator doors for weeks and even months during the school year.

First-born girls aren't often pressured quite as hard to be "crown princess," but they do wind up being in charge a lot. Older sisters are usually very dependable and conscientious, and a lot of mothers know it and take advantage of it. First-born girls often get labels like "Mother Hen" or even "The Warden."

Sometimes, however, when the girl is the oldest, she can have a good relationship with the baby in the family. This happened to me and my sister, Sally. Sally is very proud of both her brothers and as adults all three of us stay in close touch by telephone almost every week, even though we live in separate parts of the country—Sally in New York, Jack in California, and myself in Arizona.

Because Jack is closer to Sally in age, her relationship to him is one of mutual respect. With me, however, she did a lot of mothering when we were children, and she still mothers me, much to my delight. As I have been writing this book I have spent several weeks of the summer in western New York visting Sally and her family. She has already baked three raspberry and two blueberry pies—all especially for me. Of course, my own kids got most of them, but it demonstrates how my big sister is still taking care of me.

First Borns Have to Grow Up Fast

It's no wonder first borns often grow up to be serious, conscientious, and cautious. Mom and Dad have taught them to be wary of life's shoals, reefs, and rocks. At the very least they have learned to pull their oars. How often they hear, "I know your sisters and brothers are acting silly, but they're younger. I expect more from you. You have to be grown up."

It seems being more grown up is the first born's major occupation for most of his life. When first borns can't quite hack it with all these expectations, pressures, and demands, they may wind up in a counselor's office. The majority of people who seek counseling help are first-born or only-born children. They have tried their best to be conscientious, achieving, dependable, mature—in a word, perfect. The result is often frustration and a great deal of guilt.

I have counseled many first-born people who feel that they have to walk the line while the rest of the world wanders from one lane to the other without seeming to pay any consequences. It's not quite that way, of course, but when you've grown up carrying the weight of responsibility, character, and values, the load can get heavy indeed.

First borns are "first come," and they are "first served" by eager parents who want to do this job of parenting better than anyone has ever done it before. But in the long run, they are also first into the pressure cooker of life, where they have to produce or else.

What can first borns do to cope with this "curse" fate has laid upon their shoulders? As a matter of fact, they can do a great deal. But before we talk about that, I want to help first borns realize they really don't have it so bad. There's one other birth order that can make the fastidious first born look almost sloppy when it comes to being conscientious, goal oriented, and driven by the furies of perfectionism. Who can these superhuman wonderpersons be? We'll meet them in the next chapter.

Tips for First Borns Making Your Birth Order Work for You

As a first born you are quite likely a conscientious, perfectionistic, reliable person. This is a great asset, because people look up to you, trust you, and feel they can count on you. But at the same time you should be aware that your strengths can become weaknesses. Here are some tips:

1. Take smaller bites of life. First borns are known for getting themselves involved in too many things—too many activities, organizations, projects, etc. They wind up with little time for themselves.

2. Work on saying no. Many first borns are pleasers—they like the approval of others and almost always accept invitations, requests, etc.

One of the best ways to know how to say no is to know your limits. You can't do everything.

3. Remember that as a first born your parents probably had higher expectations for you than anybody else in the family. And the natural result is that you have high expectations for yourself. You expect to be first, best—perfect. Perfectionism is a great way to commit slow suicide. Lower your sights a little. Do a little less and enjoy life more.

4. First borns are known for asking a lot of questions, wanting all the details. Don't apologize for this trait, which is a sign of a leader who can size up the situation, be able to outline what has to be done, and then apply a logical, step-by-step process to solve the problem.

5. As a first born you are likely to be a cautious, careful person. Don't let people pressure you into jumping into things when you would prefer to take the time you need to make your decision.

6. If you are the serious type, try to develop a sense of humor. Learn to laugh at your mistakes. At least be more accepting of the fact that you are bound to fail now and then. Mistakes are a great way to learn and improve.

7. Never apologize for being conscientious and overorganized. As a first born you need structure; you need your "to do" lists. The trick

is not to be driven by all this. Enjoy being organized and well planned, and then share your skills with others. An awful lot of people around you could use some help!

Chapter Four

Meet Super First Born: The Lonely Only

If you rank among the only-born children on this planet, right about here you could well be muttering, "Well, it's about time. Here we are on page 79 and the only child has barely been mentioned!"

I understand that kind of reaction—particularly from a "lonely only." Only children tend to be critical—of themselves as well as others—and they are often lonely, particularly if they grew up in surroundings that offered few playmates. Because their only family contacts are essentially a mother and a father, they get plenty of adult attention, but they often have difficulty relating to their peers. This problem continues right on through life and your typical only born is known for getting along far better with people who are much older or younger.

The First Question Is "Why?"

The key question for any only-born person is this: *Why* were you an only child? It's a key question for at least two reasons. If your parents had wanted several children but could have only you, be aware that all the energy and attention that had been intended for several got poured into one—you. I call this the "special jewel" phenomenon. Only children who are special jewels often arrive when their parents are older —usually in their thirties. These special jewels can become very pampered and spoiled. They have a lifelong problem with self-centeredness because it is hard to shake the basic impression they got from their earliest recollections of Mom and Dad. Those recollections left them feeling, "I am the center of the universe."

On the other hand, you may be an only child because your parents planned for only one and stuck by their plan. You may be the result of a very structured, tightly disciplined upbringing which always demanded that you be "a little adult." This is why I will often counsel an only child who has grown into what seems to be a very together adult, who is conforming, cool, and calm. But this person is actually seething with inner rebellion. The phrase *inner rebellion* aptly describes the only child. In many cases his life has been so structured and measured out that he has a powerful current of resentment flowing just below the surface of his confident facade. Many only children grow up resenting how they always had to be such "little adults."

Only children have told me they never had a childhood. So much was expected of them that they always felt like adults. In fact, if you want a perfect description of your classic only child, use all the words I have already applied to first borns. Labels such as perfectionistic, reliable, conscientious, well-organized, critical, serious, scholarly, cautious, and conservative all apply, but preceding each label add the word *super*.

Only children—especially those who grew up in the more disciplined and structured homes— are superreliable and superconscientious. What they say they will do, they usually do. On the outside, they are very on top of things, articulate, and mature. They appear to have it all together. Yet so often, along with that inner rebellion, they feel inferior, not "up to par." The reason is that they have always been shooting for birdies and eagles. Their standards have always come from adults and have always been high—a little too high. They have never felt "quite good enough." They're always having to prove themselves again and again. This deep undercurrent of inferiority is so strong in some only children that they battle it all their lives. For many it becomes a defeating syndrome—what I call the "discouraged perfectionist," whom we will examine more closely in chapters 4 and 5.

The Special Jewel Can Be Jekyll and Hyde

Many only children can be interesting blends of oldest child and youngest child. They can be a mix of first-born characteristics and those of the last born—the baby in the family. They can act very much in charge and very adept at handling adult situations, but inside they are scared, rebellious, and angry because they have been so spoiled and pampered they are nowhere near as in control as they try to look.

This kind of only child is something of a Jekyll-Hyde personality. He is usually a "special jewel" who arrived when his parents were in their mid to late thirties, in some cases even their early forties. Some powerful forces work for and on the special jewel. Obvious, of course, is that he or she has no competition for attention from Mom and Dad. Because they had their child late in life, it is all the more precious to them. They tend to spoil the child, or at least go to great lengths to give the child all the possible advantages.

Along with the "spoiling" effect we have the fact that people who become parents late in life are more set in their ways. They have life fairly well figured. They know what they want, how they want it done, and when to do it. All this makes our special-jewel only child an excellent candidate for growing up to be an ultraperfectionist. Only children want things just so, and when things go otherwise, which is so often the case in life, they get antsy. In fact, they can get very impatient with or intolerant of people who don't measure up to their standards. Only children often quietly wish they could move in, take over, and "do it right."

Are All Only Borns Unpopular and Useless?

Life can be difficult for only-born children. One survey of college students came up with the claim that only children are perceived as more self-centered, attention seeking, unhappy, and unlikable than people with brothers and sisters.[1] This rather recent survey seems to echo the claims of Dr. Alfred Adler, who practically founded the school that stresses birth order as a critical part of psychological development. Adler made this harsh judgment on only children: "The only child has difficulties with every independent activity and sooner or later they become useless in life."[2]

While I am "adlerian" in my psychological training and approach, I have to say I think old Alfred may have had a bad day with a couple of lonely onlies when he made that statement. Plenty of only children have grown up to be quite a bit more than unhappy, unlikable, and useless. Just a few well-known only children who didn't do too badly include: Franklin D. Roosevelt, Leonardo da Vinci, the Duchess of Windsor, Charles Lindbergh, Indira Gandhi, and Albert Einstein.[3]

In my counseling work I find only children struggling far more often with perfectionism than with uselessness. I am much more likely to run across the kind of lady I will describe next. We can call her . . .

Cathy—the Discouraged Perfectionist

When the only child falls victim to perfectionism, he or she usually moves toward one of two extremes:

1. *Become very critical, cold-blooded, and objective,* never tolerating mistakes or failure on his own part or on the part of others. This person loves to go around repeating, "The good is the enemy of the best!"

2. *Become everybody's rescuer,* the one who agonizes over the problems of others and always wants to move in, take over, and solve everything. I call this the "nurse mentality" and it is no coincidence that nurses are often only children, or at least first borns in their families.

Either one of these roads can lead to becoming the one personality type I see far too much in my office—what I call the "discouraged perfectionist." Discouraged perfectionists are in fact very structured people who hold very high expectations for themselves and others. I mentioned earlier that first borns have the same trait, but only children are even more demanding in this regard.

When I suspect I have a discouraged perfectionist on my hands, I ask the client to complete a little exercise that compares the ideal self with the real self. What I'm after is to help the person contrast their "ideal" image—the self they would like to believe others see—with their "real" self—the kind of person they actually are. Below is an exhaustive version of how one person completed this assignment. Here is a comparison of the ideal and the real self by a forty-one-year-old defeated perfectionist whom I will call "Cathy."

Ideal Cathy	*Real Cathy*
organized and efficient	inefficent and unorganized
happy and cheerful	negative and grumpy
uplifting, able to bring out the best in those around me	nitpicky, discouraging to those around me
has realistic view of time and how much can be accomplished	begin things that won't fit in time slot—can't possibly finish
good housekeeper	always behind

Ideal Cathy	*Real Cathy*
able to manage household efficiently	can't get it together or get others to help
energetic and eager	mostly tired and force self to do things
sexually aggressive and expressive	tired and mechanical
realistic love expectations	unrealistic romantic—want to be pursued like before we were married
beautiful on the inside so the beauty can flow out	full of anger inside
self-confident no matter what they think	wonder what they're thinking
steady progress toward goal	procrastinate, put everything off till the last minute
finish projects	have many unfinished projects
have clean closets in home	too much clutter, can't part with anything
short and to the point	could go on and on and on
self-assured	need approval of others
feel secure	need to be needed

As I said, this is a rather exhaustive version, even for a perfectionist. For a nonperfectionist baby of the family like Leman, it was exhausting just to go over it! And Cathy said she could have gone on—and on. The above lists are the most thorough I have ever seen concerning comparison of the ideal and real person. But it doesn't surprise me; Cathy is a classic defeated perfectionist. And of course, she is an only child.

Cathy knows exactly what she is supposed to be like, but she can't measure up. Her husband, Russ, describes her as depressed, full of guilt, much too sensitive, a worrier under a lot of pressure, constantly on the go, always catching up on projects, always having to do the right thing, always biting off more than she can chew—and always feeling like a failure.

I wish you could have seen the expression on Cathy's face when I suggested that the next time she began to think discouraging thoughts, instead of coming to see me she would be money ahead to take off her high-heeled shoe and rap herself in the teeth a few times. You may have heard of the best-selling book *How to Be Your Own Best Friend.* Cathy could easily have written, *How to Be Your Own Worst Enemy.* In fact, she had several enemies living right there inside her head.

Comparing the "ideal" with the "real" helps us get to the very crux of the defeated-perfectionist personality. Actually, neither list is an accurate or healthy view of the person. On the ideal side, Cathy had set extremely high goals. When she didn't reach them, *her perception* of her real self came out as widely dissonant. She felt like a failure on every count. She really wasn't as bad as the right-hand column seemed to say. But she *thought* she was and was trapped in her own prison of unfulfilled perfectionism.

Cathy further complicated her life by having unreal expectations about marriage. We get a glimpse of this in her comparison of the ideal and the real. Notice how she felt about love and what she expected of her husband. But how realistic is it for a woman who has been married for twelve years to expect her husband to pursue her in the same way he did before they were married? I believe in romance and made a big point of how husbands should romance their wives in a book I wrote called *Sex Begins in the Kitchen,* but you can expect too much and life just doesn't work out that way.

But this was Cathy's forte—getting her hopes high, and then having her husband, Russ, fall short of her expectations. But instead of judging Russ, she turned the evidence on herself and became all the more convicted of not being a good person. Whenever Russ didn't measure up to her lofty expectations for a husband, she didn't tell herself Russ was terrible; she told herself she was terrible and if she could be a better person, Russ would behave differently!

Cathy's Father Was a Flaw Finder

You may have guessed by now that Cathy—an only child—grew up in a family with a very detached father who would never praise her for anything. In fact, he was very good at finding her flaws. Cathy always felt as if she had to measure up, but she never could, no matter how hard she tried.

For example, at age thirteen she single-handedly built a brick wall that went around the back of her home and encircled a small bricked-in patio. It was a major job for anyone and practically impossible for a thirteen-year-old girl. But in her own immature way, she pulled it off and it was an exceptionally good job. Everyone who saw the wall marveled at what she had done—except her father. When he came home from a business trip and found the wall (which he was going to get around to building someday) already up, he was enraged. Everything Cathy had done was wrong. He couldn't find one thing right with the wall or with her.

Things were bad enough growing up, but guess what kind of husband Cathy happened to marry? Russ was smart, good at his job, and very successful. But he was also a first-born child, very insecure because he always felt as if he couldn't quite measure up, either. So, it followed that he had a very critical, flaw-finding nature. On top of that, he wanted to avoid conflict.

Russ was absolutely inept at providing what Cathy really wanted in life: a husband who could share intimate thoughts and feelings with her.

So, part of the therapy program was to bring Russ in to work with him and help him learn to articulate his feelings. It was a revelation to him as he became aware that he was full of feelings but had just never learned to let them out. He had always quietly "disapproved" of Cathy and she had sensed it. When they finally got to talking, a lot of things cleared up fast.

Of course the reason behind Russ's reluctance to share feelings was that he was afraid if he ever told his wife how he felt, she would reject him. This is a classic characteristic in people whom I call "controllers." These people keep their feelings inside and have a hard time sharing them because they're afraid if they ever do they'll be rejected. It was exceptionally gratifying to help Cathy and Russ find out they could share feelings with each other and love each other just the way they were.

Another important part of Cathy's therapy was getting her to learn the word *no*. She had an overwhelming propensity to bite off more than she could chew. I had to battle with her to commit herself to weed things out of her life that were really too much for her. One of these areas included her church activities. Cathy was a very active Christian and totally committed to her church. She served on every possible board she could find. In addition, she had decided to teach her two children at home (in what is called "home school") and hold down a part-time job of some twenty-two hours a week!

There was, of course, no way Cathy could do all this very satisfactorily. She had no time for herself, not to mention time for Russ. But it was her style and she drove herself to the brink. She went around wondering if she would ever catch up. My general prescription for Cathy was to "drop some things or drop dead yourself."

I got her to agree to give up teaching her kids at home, as well as quit her part-time job. I also suggested she cut back on some of her church work, where she was doing far more than one person should. It was extremely difficult for Cathy to resign any of her positions at the church because God meant a great deal to her. But I tried to sell her on the idea that if she were really going to serve God well, she had to start by serving her husband and family in a much better fashion. I also wanted her to start treating herself better.

As an only child, Cathy was good at following directions and she became one of my "star clients." She made many changes in her life and some of them centered around backing off and saying no to a world that was constantly urging her to "go ahead and go for it." Before she sought help, Cathy was headed for a life of feeling useless and unsuccessful, exactly what Alfred Adler had said about only children years ago. But interestingly enough, while Adler could be very negative about only children, he could be very positive in other respects. For example, Adler also said that it isn't important where you were born in the family! Your particular birth order only means you have had a certain environment in which to develop. As an adult you can recognize your characteristics and take practical steps to emphasize your strong points and strengthen your weak ones.[4]

That's exactly what Cathy did! She proved there is *always* hope, even for an only child whose unfeeling father turned her into a totally discouraged perfectionist. In fact, there are so many things perfectionistic first borns and only children can do to combat perfectionism that I have devoted the entire next chapter to just that. Perfectionists from other birth orders are also welcome. As a hang-loose "baby" of the family (and anything but a perfectionist) I believe it's vital to learn how to try to be less than perfect— and be a lot happier.

Tips for Only Children
Making Your Birth Order Work for You

Because only children are "first borns in triplicate," all of the tips on pages 76 and 77 are applicable here. Superconscientious and reliable only children should pay close attention, however, to several points:

1. Be ruthless with yourself in regard to making too many commitments and expecting too much of yourself. It is all too easy to reach the point where every day is a rat race, with no end in sight.

2. Is time and space for yourself really built into your schedule? Most only children are the type who need some time for themselves. Make sure it happens.

3. As a rule, only children get along better with people much older or much younger than themselves. You can't control the ages of everyone you work with or deal with, but in some cases you can try to arrange experiences with people who are older or younger. Do it, because these are personalities you are more likely to click with. These are the people who will give you more strokes and argue with you less.

4. Only children are often labeled selfish and self-centered because they never had to learn to share with brothers and sisters. Take some hon-

93

est inventory of your own life. How self-centered do you act around your spouse, friends, or fellow workers? What specific things can you do to put others first, help others more, and be less critical of others?

Chapter Five

Prescription for Discouraged Perfectionists

CHRISTIAN, blond, blue eyes, 5'2", 100 lbs. prof., cauc/female, no depend., wishes to meet Protestant Christian, prof. man in 30s with college degree who has compassion for animals and people, loves nature, exercise and phy. fitness (no team sports), music and dance, church and home life. Desire nonsmoker/ nondrinker, slender, 5'7"–6', lots of head hair, no chest hair, intelligent, honest and trustworthy, sense of humor, excellent communicator of feelings, very sensitive, gentle, affectionate, androgynous attitude about roles, giving, encouraging and helpful to others, no temper or ego problems, secure within and financially, health conscious, neat and clean, extremely considerate and dependable. I believe in old-fashioned morals and values. If you do too, and are interested in a possible Christian commitment, write to PO Box 82533. Please include recent color photo and address.

I don't know what you make of the above want ad, which I clipped right out of a daily newspaper, but it tells me one thing: The odds are at least 500 to 1 that this blond, blue-eyed, 5′2″, 100 lb. female is a first-born (or quite possibly an only-born) child. I can't help but wonder what this superperfectionist lady would do if some superman answered her ad and qualified at every point except one—he had a lot of hair on his chest! Or what would she do if the poor guy wanted to play on the church softball team (no team sports, remember!). We can only hope that she would be willing to give in at a few points. If not, it's likely that our blue-eyed blond will grow old alone, waiting for Mr. Right to call.

Little Things Drive Perfectionists Crazy

The reason I'm so sure a first born or only child placed the above ad is that it is a classic example of the kind of expectations and demands a perfectionist will display in life. If I have to single out one word to describe first borns or only children, it has to be *perfectionistic.* It's almost as though they have inner forces working on them that are hard to control. At least that seems to be the case with our daughter, Holly. I vowed to never let my first born fall into the perfectionist's pit. Well, Sande and I tried, we really did, but perhaps I should have seen the handwriting on the wall—more correctly, the sand—when we took eighteen-month-old Holly along for a little R & R trip to California and the seashore. It was Holly's first time on any beach and she proceeded to discover sand. She came toddling over and held up one finger with three or four grains of sand stuck to it.

"Ugh, ugh," she grunted, obviously most displeased with the mess and wondering what we were going to do about it.

I resisted the temptation to give a brief fatherly lecture such as, "Yes, Holly, the fact is this: If you're on the beach, you're going to have sand stick somewhere on your body." But I should have realized right then, that even at eighteen months, Holly was displaying signs of the true perfectionist. Now, at age twelve, she has definitely become just that. Despite our efforts to encourage and reinforce her rather than find fault or pick flaws, Holly seeks perfection. If things don't go exactly right in life, she gets frustrated, even edgy. It's the little things, not the really big things, that bother the perfectionists of this world. Little things, like a few grains of sand, a smudge on a paper, or leaving two minutes late, really drive a perfectionist crazy.

Can a Slob Be a Perfectionist?

I realize I'm assuming a lot when I say all first borns and only children are perfectionists, and critics often challenge me with examples that seem to totally contradict that idea: "You don't know my husband, Harry. He's an only child and a total slob. The only thing he has ever perfected is making a mess."

"You should live with my wife, Gertrude. She's a first born but the only way I can get her anywhere on time is to tell her we are due anywhere from thirty to sixty minutes earlier than the actual appointment."

I still say Harry and Gertrude are almost certainly perfectionists. They are, however, the kind who mask their perfectionism with behavior that doesn't seem to fit. They are in the select but unfortunate group called "discouraged perfectionists."

Perfectionists go through life telling themselves the lie, "I only count when I'm perfect." If you want a heavy burden to carry around, just take that one on. Everything the perfectionist does must be right. What a price he pays for convincing himself, "I only count when I'm perfect." And when he starts believing that lie, he joins the ranks of the *discouraged* perfectionists— those driven souls who hate mistakes and errors but still have to make the best of it. Discouraged perfectionists may act out of character—be sloppy, for example—but it is all a cover to hide their frustration with life's less-than-perfect warts and bumps.

It's interesting that stutterers tend to be first-born children. When you encounter a stutterer, you're usually talking to a perfectionist. In other words, the fear of making a mistake is so great that it impedes the stutterer's natural ability to talk. He fears making a mistake, so what does he do? He makes mistakes.

Perfectionists Are Skillful Procrastinators

Many discouraged perfectionists really have difficulties in handling time. They're the expert procrastinators who sometimes do a little bit and then walk away from the task. They seem to be "either or" kind of people. When they're running hot, watch out. They'll trample you getting all that work done. But when they're running cold, it's tough to get them to move at all.

Procrastinators tend to be stubborn people. The mood has to be just right or they can't possibly hit on all eight cylinders. Naturally, they have high expectations for their own performance, and this means they often drive themselves wacky with details. They're the ones who stay up until two in the morning looking for the ten cents they're missing in the checking account. Babies in the family, like me, could be down a thousand and it wouldn't matter. We would go to bed by ten o'clock.

I recently counseled a man who had not filed his income tax forms for the last four years. Why hadn't he filed? He had such an elaborate system for keeping records and receipts that reporting his income tax became an insurmountable task. His family room contained several picnic tables, nicely covered with shelf paper, all overflowing with neatly stacked piles of receipts, notes, and bills of sale.

This man had a way of lying to himself. The lie was that he was totally dedicated to details and getting things right. But all he was doing was prohibiting himself from enjoying life by always having something hanging over his head. And I really can't think of anything worse to have hanging over your head than the IRS. And the final irony was that the government owed *him* some money!

It's not surprising that this man had a critical wife who was always asking him to do things around the house. "George, when are you going to fix the toaster?" And George would say, "Don't worry, Alice, I'll do it tomorrow." And as you could predict, tomorrow would come and the toaster never got fixed.

Poor George ended up with so many uncompleted tasks staring him in the face that he essentially was kept in the position of treading water in the swimming pool of life. He wasn't moving toward the shallow end of the pool and he wasn't moving toward the deep end, either. He wasn't swimming any laps—he was simply treading water.

Of course, you can't tread water forever. Sooner or later you've got to get moving and commit yourself one way or another.

After quite a few sessions I finally got George to attack his problems one at a time. I got him to where he could take care of the toaster on Monday and then try fixing the doorjamb on Tuesday. The commitment he had to make was that he couldn't start project B until project A got done. That's always the key to the discouraged perfectionist. He has to commit himself to do one thing before he starts another. This all sounds rather simple, I know, but this one basic principle can do wonders if the person has the commitment to carry it through. To paraphrase the old saying, "Tomorrow may never come—do it now, one step at a time."

Perfectionists Pummel Themselves and One Another

Because discouraged perfectionists are often stubborn, opinionated, and strong willed, they become known for telling people exactly what they think. And what happens if you tell everyone what you think? You drive them away. You lose your friends. Even your enemies don't want to hang around long enough to try to insult you.

When the discouraged perfectionist is told he's too outspoken, he says, "Okay, fine . . . I'll just keep everything inside. If you guys can't handle it, I won't say anything."

And then what happens? The perfectionist loses his health. Any time you have anxiety in your life (and it can be conscious or unconscious), that anxiety will come out somewhere, somehow. It will be manifested in certain parts of your body. That's why the large number of people who go to see psychologists when they have migraines, stomach disorders, backaches, etc., are generally first-born or only children. They're the worriers of life, the ones who develop colitis, ulcers, facial tics, and cluster headaches.

What Can the Discouraged Perfectionist Do?

Following are some suggestions I have seen work wonders in the lives of perfectionists.

1. *First and foremost, realize that perfectionism is a deadly enemy.* I call it "slow suicide." Only children are the worst offenders, followed by first borns. I've seen later-born children who were perfectionists, also.

Actually, *perfectionism* has a couple of definitions. It might mean being best at everything you try, which is usually the male's approach because he needs to achieve. Or it could mean being as complete and thorough as you possibly can be, which is more typically a female approach designed to avoid criticism.[1]

To control your perfectionism, you must recognize your desperate need to be perfect. Not only that, you must recognize the fallacy and futility in this kind of thinking. You are *never* going to be perfect. Why not give yourself permission to be imperfect? Do it just for today. Don't worry about tomorrow. Tomorrow will come soon enough.

Start each day by giving yourself permission to be imperfect. Make a conscious effort to go easy on criticizing yourself and others. In fact, it may be easier to start with others. When someone makes a mistake, try to separate the deed from the doer, never an easy task. Keep in mind, if you have to give somebody feedback (particularly your children), that person will have a hard time separating your criticism of what he did from his own self-image. Practice talking about what happened instead of saying, *"You* did this," or *"You* did that."

It also helps to realize that leopards don't change their spots. The "spots" in your mate or your children are not going to go away. Our tendency is to say, "I want my husband, or my wife, or my teenager, to change and *I'm* going to see that it happens." Well, good luck. You may have heard it before but it's strange how often I have to say it in counseling sessions: *There is no way you can change anybody else's behavior.* You can only change your own behavior and when you do make a genuine effort to do that, the strangest thing can happen. It allows other people in your life to make the behavioral changes you've been hoping for!

2. *Memorize this three-word sentence and use it often: "I was wrong."* As you make progress on this one, try two more that are just as difficult: "I'm sorry" and "Will you forgive me?"

These three short sentences total nine words in all. They could be the toughest nine words to utter in any language. They are particularly hard for perfectionists, but they are also a ticket to freedom from the chains of frustration. Memorize and use these nine words and you will learn that it is okay to fail.

3. *Don't be so quick to put yourself down, and when others criticize, don't be so quick to react.* Perfectionists are *sensitive.* Be aware of your sensitivity. Admit it and cope with it. How? Realize that time is on your side. It takes time to change ingrained patterns.

For example, watch for those times when you catch yourself being very sensitive or defensive about a criticism, whether it comes from others or from within yourself. You won't always be able to anticipate these times and head them off. Often you may have to look back in retrospect and say, "Yes, I really didn't need to get so upset yesterday when I forgot to mail that important letter." But even becoming aware after the fact is still progress. I repeat, ingrained patterns are not changed overnight.

One practical suggestion I give sensitive perfectionists is this: "Do nice things for yourself." As the hair color ad says, "You're worth it."

But it isn't always easy to convince perfectionists that they are worth it. I remember working with a client several years ago who used to go to the local department store, buy some new clothes, and then return them a few days later. This woman was a class A perfectionist who *always* returned whatever she bought because invariably something just wasn't quite right. The psychological message I got from this behavior was that she didn't think she was worth the new clothes. She was telling herself, "You aren't worth a new dress. You don't deserve a new sweater."

But this woman really needed new clothes. She hadn't bought herself anything new for several years. That is, she bought clothes but she didn't keep them. I finally got her to see that it would be okay to buy something new and keep it. She didn't have to find fault with something she was getting for herself. She was worth that new dress!

4. *Perfectionists often overwhelm themselves with the BIG PICTURE.* They take on too much at once. So, work at doing one thing at a time. Finish A before tackling B. I realize that some things come up—phone calls, for example, interrupt the major report you start at 9:00 A.M. The point is, don't start a major report at 9:00 A.M. and then schedule a major meeting at 9:30.

Also, as you schedule things, take a hard look at your expectations. Perfectionists are famous for unrealistic expectations and setting goals that are far too high.

5. *Right along with becoming more skilled in scheduling and goal setting is the need to become skilled in saying no.* As I have said so many times, perfectionists tend to be first borns and only children. And what do we know about these people? They want and need the approval of others. It's very difficult for them to say, "No, I can't do that," or "No, I don't want to do that."

And so the perfectionist gets trapped in many situations where he says yes when he really wants to say no. Not being able to say no can raise a person's frustration level to the point where he is literally ready to explode.

If you can't learn to say no to people, you will never be able to say yes to life. There are just too many people who will take advantage and pull you in a dozen different directions to get what they want. Very often you will find these people in your very own family. But if you constantly find yourself unable to say no, it usually means saying yes to headaches and stomach problems.

6. *Perfectionists are often pessimists.* Work on seeing the proverbial glass as half full, not half empty. Positive thinking is more than the topic for best-selling books by Dr. Norman Vincent Peale. It is one of the most powerful psychological forces on earth. Use it.

For example, think about and meditate on things you are thankful for. More important, think about people you are thankful for and why. Remind yourself of three good things that happened today—or maybe last week. Then think about what can happen during the coming week that will be pleasing and pleasant.

7. *First borns and only children often have trouble sharing their thoughts and feelings, even with themselves.* Why? Because they fear if they tell someone what they really think (admit who they really are) that person will reject them.

The best person to start sharing your thoughts and feelings with is yourself. Change negative self-talk to positive self-talk. For example, instead of saying, "I hate these kinds of meetings," say, "I usually don't like these meetings, but this time I am looking forward to it."

Instead of saying, "I'll make a fool of myself," say, "I'm not afraid of doing anything foolish. The other people there are not judging me."

Instead of saying, "I can't talk in front of

groups," say, "I usually don't like to talk to groups, but I am prepared and what I have to say is important."[2]

8. *One other tip about relating to others: Perfectionists aren't known for being forgiving.* In fact, when insulted or unappreciated, they can nurse grudges for far too long. Do you need to work on your ability to grant forgiveness? For the perfectionist, the key to forgiveness lies in realizing that people make mistakes and the world still goes on.

It all comes back to what was said earlier about authority and living by the letter of the law. In my counseling I find that the typical view first borns and only children have of God is that He is a judge, policeman, or at best a referee who is trying to keep the game honest. A major cause for this kind of perception is the first-born or only-born person's relationship to the parents, especially the father. He grows up with adults as primary role models and, of course, he buys into authority and authority figures rather thoroughly.

When I counsel I often notice only children and first borns having difficulty with the concept of God's grace and forgiveness. When first borns and only children pray, they tend to address God by using what I call their "ideal self." That is, they pray according to how they would like to be or how they want the world to see them.

An ideal-self kind of prayer sounds like this: "Lord, please help me be more tolerant of little Buford, or my husband, or whoever." The ideal-self prayer shies away from getting down to the *real me* and telling it like it is: "Lord, I have a lousy temper. Forgive me for the way I chewed out my family today."

First borns and only children have this dissonance between their real selves and their ideal selves because they tend to rely too much on their own abilities. They believe in God, but act as though He really isn't big enough to forgive them. They almost seem to want to control God. They decide what God can forgive and what He can't, or they get hung up on thinking they have to *do* something to earn His forgiveness.

Don't Let Life Blow Out Your Candle

One counseling technique I use quite often is to ask adults to give me between five and ten very early recollections of their lives. These may be only faint memories or brief glimpses, but they mean something. They wouldn't have stuck there in the memory for all these years if they didn't. I believe these early recollections are consistent with the way a person sees life today. I will even go a step further and say that the first recollections of life are usually symbolic of a person's entire life-style.

I once worked with a young man in his twenties whose first recollections of life included looking out the window and watching the other boys flying kites in a stiff breeze. It seemed to him that ever since he was small, he had been standing on the sidelines watching other people have fun. And when he came to me, he was still in that state—basically watching life go by and not doing much with his potential. He just wasn't getting involved and he was always wishing he was like others whom he admired or envied.

Guess this young man's birth order. Of course —he was the oldest child. And guess what his parents were like—you're right, they were overly perfectionistic and overdemanding. They blew out his candle at an early age. He simply lacked the self-confidence to try much of anything.

Now obviously all first borns and only children don't wind up as this young man did. But I think his story is symbolic of one of the real pressures that face your first- or only-born children. They have so much going for them: ambition, strong powers of concentration, excellent organizational and planning skills, original creative thinking. They are precise in their thinking and have excellent memories. They usually come across as leaders and are looked up to by the rest of society. They have it together.

But all of this can get out of balance, and the

imbalanced state is perfectionism. Perfectionists really have to work at being open, tolerant, and patient—with others and themselves. They can't accomplish this in a weekend seminar or by reading one or two books. It's a lifelong task.

I believe that few only-born children ever completely lick their propensity to be intolerant and impatient toward the mere mortals with whom they have to live. But over the years any first-born or only-born person can mature and grow emotionally and spiritually. It wouldn't hurt for every first- and only-born person to own two or three T-shirts that say: "I must learn to be patient with myself and others—God isn't finished with us yet!"

The Difference Between Being Excellent and Being Perfect

With all this critiquing of perfectionism, you may be wondering what happened to the pursuit of excellence. Must first borns and only children in particular drop their standards in order to live happily? Not if they understand the difference between trying to be perfect and trying to be excellent:

Perfectionists
reach for impossible goals

Pursuers of Excellence
enjoy meeting high standards that are within reach

Perfectionists	Pursuers of Excellence
value themselves by what they do	value themselves by who they are
get depressed and give up	may experience disappointment, but keep going
are devastated by failure	learn from failure
remember mistakes and dwell on them	correct mistakes, then learn from them
can only live with being number one	are happy with being number two, if they know they have tried their hardest
hate criticism	welcome criticism
have to win to keep high self-esteem	finish second and still have a good self-image

Part Three

Later Borns and How They Tick

If you came after the first born in the family you're either a middle child or a last born (baby). Being born later in the family has its perks—and its problems. In the next two chapters you'll learn . . .

- why middle children become master negotiators
- which birth order is the best bet to stay in a marriage
- why last borns develop an "I'll show them" attitude
- the birth order you find most often in car sales
- the ingredient that keeps the last born going indefinitely
- why middle children often feel squeezed out at home

- why later borns are less fearful than first borns
- which birth order is the last to seek help
- which birth order is hardest to spot
- who is most likely to spoil the annual family photo

Chapter Six

Middle Child: Born Too Late . . . and Too Soon

Like the title of this chapter, the middle child is a bit mysterious. I counsel adults who grew up as middle children (that is, somewhere between the first born and the last born) and as they share their frustrations, the classic pattern usually emerges. They were born *too late* to get the privileges and special treatment the first born seemed to inherit by right. And they were born *too soon* to strike the bonanza that many last borns enjoy —the relaxing of the disciplinary reins, which is sometimes translated into "getting away with murder."

Perhaps no birth order specialists put it better than Bradford Wilson and George Edington in *First Child, Second Child* when they say that of all birth order positions, middleness is the most difficult to define, let alone describe or generalize about in any meaningful way.[1]

I agree with Wilson and Edington that the middle born just isn't as easy to spot and define as people who are youngest or oldest in their families. Keep in mind that the term *middle* can mean many things. Perhaps the typical middle child is the second of three, but he could also be the third of four, the fourth of five children, and so on. Some textbooks go into great detail on the various kinds of middle-born children. In my counseling, however, I discovered that middle children and second borns have a great deal in common, and are often one and the same because so many families stop at three. For our purposes in this chapter we will group the second born and middle child together and simply call them "middle children." In chapter 12 we will take a special look at parenting the two-child family and the dynamics at work when number two arrives to give number one his or her first taste of competition for the attentions of Mom and Dad.

One Word for Middle Borns Is "Contradictions"

Whenever you deal with the middle children of the family you have to consider the "branching-off effect" that has been at work. This principle says the second born will be most directly influenced by the first born, the third born will be most directly influenced by the second born, and so on. By "influence" I mean that each child looks above and sizes up the older sibling. For example, the second born has the first born for his role model and as he perceives the first born in action, the second born develops a style of life of his own. If he senses he can compete with the older sibling, he may do so. But if the older brother or sister is stronger, smarter, etc., the second born typically shoots off in another direction.

The thing to remember is that any time a second-born child enters the family, his life-style will be determined by his perception. He might be a pleaser or an antagonizer. He might become a victim or a martyr. He might become a manipulator or a controller. Any number of life-styles can appear, but *they all play off the first born.* For example, if the first born is a perfectly compliant little fellow, that second-born son might really be a handful. The general conclusion of all research studies done on birth order is that second borns will probably be somewhat the opposite of first borns.

Because later-born children "bounce off" the ones directly above them, there is no way to predict which way they might go or how their personalities might develop. Characteristic charts on middle-born children often sound like an exercise in paradoxical futility. For example, below are two columns with words and phrases that can all be very typical of the middle child. It's not hard to spot the direct contradictions:

loner, quiet, shy	sociable, friendly, outgoing
impatient, easily frustrated	takes life in stride, laid back
very competitive	easygoing—not competitive
rebel, family goat	peacemaker, mediator
aggressive, a scrapper	avoids conflict

The middle child is "iffy"—the product of many pressures coming from different directions. You must always look at the entire family to understand the plight of the middle child. How he finally turns out is about as predictable as a Chicago weather report. In many ways, the middle child remains a mystery.

Middle Kids Just Don't Get Much Respect

While the middle child's characteristics are not always easy to predict, something else is. The middle child always feels the "squeeze" from above and below. Was Rodney Dangerfield a middle child? It's likely. Many middle children would identify with Rodney's famous lament and agree: "I just didn't get much respect!"

As I have counseled middle-born children, they have often told me they did not feel that special growing up. The first born had his place and the baby of the family had his special spot, but the middle child? There just didn't seem to be that much room or even a great deal of parental awareness of the need for a spot on the pecking order. The following scene is fictitious, but it is all too true for many middle borns:

> When Mama introduced Sylvie, she always said, "This is Sylvie, my oldest child."
> When Mama introduced Rufus, she always said, "This is Rufus, the baby in the family."
> When Mama introduced Joey to people, she would say, "This is Joey, my oldest son."
> But when Mama introduced Jane, she just said, "This is Jane." Because Mama had not figured out that Jane was the middle Moffat. Nobody had figured this out, but Jane.[2]

One of the telltale signs that Mom and Dad sort of relegate the middle child to the background is the family photo album. If I want to get a rise out of second-born children in particular at a seminar, all I have to say is, "Family photo album." They laugh, but often a bit sardonically. The typical story reveals two thousand pictures of the first born and thirteen of them. Second-born children in particular seem to fall victim to the strange phenomenon. It is almost as if Mom and Dad suddenly went on welfare and couldn't buy any film, or the camera got broken and wasn't fixed until "baby princess" came along.

Picture (no pun intended) the scene. A thirteen-year-old girl falls in puppy love for the first time and wants to give her photo to her boyfriend. She goes to her mother and says, "Hey, Mom, are there any pictures of me without *her?*" Mom looks a little chagrined and has to shake her head no. So, the new boyfriend gets his photo—carefully trimmed so older sister's armpit barely shows!

Fifth Wheels Need All the Friends They Can Get

It's no surprise to find middle-born children who feel as if they were fifth wheels out of place, misunderstood, or just some kind of leftover who always got bypassed and upstaged by the younger or older siblings. That's why it's not unusual for middle-born children to hang out more with their peer group than any other child in the family. Friends become very important to the middle-born child. At home, the first born is special because he or she is first. The last born is special because he or she means the end of the line. But the middle child is "just plain Mary" or "good old John."

There is a psychological theory that says human beings operate according to three natural motivations:

1. To obtain rewards and recognition.
2. To avoid pain and danger.
3. To get even.[3]

Every birth order has these three motivations operating in life, but it is especially interesting to trace their effect on the behavior of the typical middle born.

To obtain reward and recognition, the squeezed-out middle born goes outside the family to create another kind of "family" where he or she can feel special. First borns typically have fewer friends. Middle children often have many.

"How sad," you might say, "that the middle-born child has to go outside the family to get recognition and feelings of acceptance." But weep not for our social butterfly. All these relationships will pay off later, as I'll explain in a moment.

So, to avoid the pain and frustration of being an "outsider" in his family, the middle child "leaves home" the quickest. I don't mean he runs away or volunteers for boarding school, but he makes friends more quickly at school and in the neighborhood. Tired of being told, "You're too young," when he seeks the same privileges as the oldest, and weary of hearing, "You're too old," when he whines for a little TLC like that

121

given the youngest, the middle child goes where he is "just the right age"—to his peer group.

And, to get even, at least a little bit for those feelings of rootlessness, the middle child becomes a bit of a "free spirit." He gives himself the right to reject the family's do's and don'ts, at least in part, by choosing some other group's values for a measuring stick. It may be a team (middle children are great team players), a club, or a gang of kids who hang out together. The important thing is that the middle child experiences the group *as his,* something his family can't control or squeeze in any way.

Middle Children Become Good Mediators

Of course, some middle children choose other ways to meet their needs for obtaining recognition, avoiding pain, and getting even. They may prefer becoming mediators and even at times be manipulative. Because they couldn't have Mom and Dad all to themselves and get their way, they learn to negotiate and compromise. And again, these obviously aren't such bad skills to have for getting along later in life. (If you are getting the message that middle children just might turn out to be the best-adjusted adults in the family, you're right, but more on that later.)

The middle child's propensity to negotiate

and compromise can backfire, however. An attractive, nicely dressed woman will come to me for counseling. It will turn out that she's been married to her husband for anywhere from twenty to thirty years and they have raised several children. The woman is a second born and she has been something of a superwife and supermom.

After a couple of sessions, the truth comes out: Her husband has been having affairs throughout their marriage. He is probably having an affair at that very time, undoubtedly with a younger, more attractive woman. But the second-born wife is sticking it out—again. She is following her basic life-style, which had her growing up to be a pleaser, very much against rocking the boat, wanting the oceans of life to be as smooth as possible.

True, part of her endurance comes from her love for her husband and her family, but a great part of her motivation is her need to have peace at just about any price. The wife is hurting; she comes to a counselor for help but the pattern is set. Many courses of action are open to her: move out, serve papers, confront the other woman, tell the children—in general, force her husband's hand. But she doesn't really want to do anything. She is a victim and she indulges in what is called victim thinking. She will hang tough with her cheating hubby until the bitter end, and he knows it.

How to Stand Your Middle Ground

As you can see, it's hard to come up with as clear a composite picture of middle children as you can with first borns or only children. But here are some observations and suggestions that can help the adult middle child function with better understanding of himself and how he relates to others:

1. *Studies show middle children are the most secretive of all the birth orders.*[4] If this applies to you, realize you could be displaying what psychologists call the "burned child" reaction. The burned child experiences the world as paying him less attention than it did his older or younger brothers or sisters. As a result, you may play it "closer to the vest" in your relationships and choose not to confide in very many people. This isn't necessarily serious, except possibly in marriage, where you can come up with little or no communication, something we will give a close look in Part Four.

2. *Middle children prove to be the last to seek the services of helping professions such as psychologists, counselors, or ministers.*[5] Who shows up more often in my office? First-born engineers, doctors —people in professions that are demanding and exacting. They analyze their plight and seek the help of an "authority" who can fix it. The next largest group to come are last borns—the babies who are used to being cared for and helped. I

see fewer middle children, but that is not too difficult to understand. It can be the burned-child reaction coming out (or is the burned child hiding?). And it can also be the mental toughness and independence the middle child acquires while learning to cope with feelings of rejection and "fifth wheelness" while growing up at home.

It's fine to be tough and independent, but it's foolish to refuse to get the kind of help you need. If you find yourself in a situation where you just might need some counseling, sit down and think things through. You might be cutting off your nose to spite your face with an "I'll show them" attitude that you got way back on that day when your older sister got to go to the beach and you didn't and a couple of hours later you got grounded for a month when you slugged your little brother for being such a pest.

3. *Middle-born children are known, of course, for "running with the pack," especially as teenagers.* [6] Did you give your mom and dad fits by going along with what they thought was the wrong crowd? If so, you should have good insight into why your own children may be doing the same thing.

I counsel many families where the parents are worried about a child who seems to be "running with the wrong crowd." If the child is a middle born, I try to help them see the forces that may be at work. More on this in Part Five.

4. *Middle-born children are considered the most monogamous of all birth orders.* [7] This makes sense. They didn't feel they fit in that well while growing up. When they start their own family, they have a strong desire to make the marriage work. This is an excellent quality but it can lead to a lot of pain for one spouse when the other takes advantage by being unfaithful, abusive, or dominating.

5. *Middle-born children are prone to embarrassment, but they will never admit it.* [8] That figures. Admitting it would be too embarrassing! This is part of that middle-born tendency to be a contradiction. Middle borns are often a bit rebellious as far as convention is concerned, but at the same time they never want to look unsophisticated—what the younger generation calls "not cool."

To sum it up, the middle is really not such a bad spot. All the research shows that middle-born children don't have as many hang-ups or problems as first borns or only children. If you are a middle born you may think that your big brother or sister got all the breaks and privileges while you were growing up. But there's more to life than getting breaks and privileges. Studies show that later-born children are less fearful and anxious than first borns. Why? Because first borns sense the fear and anxiety in the new parents who are wrestling with problems and crises they never experienced before. By the time the parents had number two, they were more relaxed. Also, the middle child has the benefit of having his first-born sibling "run interference" for him—what I like to call snowplowing the roads of life a bit.

It's interesting that Alfred Adler, father of birth order psychology, believed that in most cases being the middle child was a fairly safe spot, although Adler did admit the second born with a brilliant older brother or sister could be in for trouble. But even if you had to live in the shadow of a brilliant crown prince or princess, don't waste time on self-pity. Be thankful for the experience, which at least gives you empathy for people who don't always get to be the star.

Kathy Nessel, a psychologist colleague and a middle child herself, sums up the "advantages" of middledom this way: "Middle children are tenacious adults because we are used to life being rather unfair. Our expectations are lower: consequently we are more accepting in a relationship. The middle child may say, 'Well, this isn't perfect, but it is kind of nice.' We are not as driven as first borns, but then again, neither are we as compulsive."[9]

Perhaps a good description of middle children is "balanced." And in this topsy-turvy world, balanced is not a bad way to fly. As one middle child told me recently, "Being a middle child of three wasn't easy, but as an adult I really believe I can cope with problems better because I got a lot of good training in give-and-take while I was growing up. I'm glad I wasn't first and I'm glad I wasn't last. I'm glad I'm me!"

Tips for Middle Borns
Making Your Birth Order Work for You

In books on birth order, the middle child sometimes comes off as someone to be pitied. Hand-me-downs, fewer photos in the family album, and feeling like an outsider or fifth wheel are all the stereotyped fates of the middle child. But while first borns and last borns get more attention, I believe middle children get better training for life. Instead of feeling deprived, the middle child should make the most of the tools he or she has gained while growing up.

1. You probably have certain people-oriented social skills because of all the negotiating and mediating you had to do while growing up. Use these skills to see both sides and deal with life as it really is.

2. You may be saying, "I'm really not much of a negotiator—really I'm more of a free spirit —I like to do my thing." Keep in mind that if anybody is unpredictable, it's a middle child. If you are the free-spirit type, fight to keep your unique qualities. Keep in mind that businesses

and companies are often looking for someone with new ideas and the independence to try them.

3. Middle children may sometimes grow up telling themselves that their family never listened to them so no one else will listen to them, either. Instead of apologizing for your opinions, or failing to offer them at all, share your ideas with others. You'll be amazed at how many people are looking for someone who doesn't want to do *all the taking!*

4. If the "socially skilled, lots of friends" label fits you, rejoice and enjoy it. But don't spread yourself too thin. No one can maintain a limitless number of relationships and keep them meaningful.

5. Don't get sucked in to playing comparison games. You understand better than anyone that there are always people who are above or below in terms of ability, interest, appearance, athletic skill, etc. Comparisons are futile and usually pointless. Just be comfortable with being you.

6. Don't get the mistaken idea that first borns are the only people who can rise to positions of leadership. Middle children often make excellent managers and leaders becuase they understand compromise, negotiation, and giving something for something else (the art of quid pro quo). If you are in a position right now

where you can try for a manager's slot, don't hesitate because you think you don't have enough charisma, dynamic, etc. Use your natural middle-child skills to go for it!

Chapter Seven

Family Baby: Born Last but Seldom Least

The year is 1952. The scene is a hot, sweaty gymnasium at Williamsville Central High School in western New York. A hard-fought basketball game is in progress and a skinny little eight-year-old kid is out on the floor during a time-out trying to lead cheers. Pinned on his sweater is an image of the team mascot—a billy goat.

The game is as close as the air. The place is packed with screaming fans but at the moment the fans aren't screaming for their "Billies." They're all laughing at this little kid, who has gotten the cheer completely backwards and forgotten what comes next. His big sister, captain of the Williamsville cheerleaders, looks embarrassed, but she has to laugh, too, because this little kid is pretty funny.

But is the little eight-year-old guy embarrassed? He doesn't seem to mind at all. In fact, he is looking up at the crowd and kind of enjoying the fact they are all laughing!

Last Borns Often Love the Limelight

I was that little kid—born last in a batch of three. I have already introduced you to Sally and Jack, born first and second, the real lions of the Leman clan. And then came last-born Kevin, who got the nickname "Cub" when he was eleven days old. The name stuck and as I became a toddler and a preschooler I instinctively became aware of how to always be "cute little Cubby" in the family. The youngest may have been born last, but he has a sixth sense that tells him he's not going to be least!

Youngest children in the family are typically the outgoing charmers, the personable manipulators. They are also affectionate, uncomplicated, and sometimes a little absentminded. Their "space cadet" approach to life gets laughs, smiles, and shakes of the head. Last borns are the most likely to show up at the elementary school's "sing" or the Sunday-school picnic unzipped or unbuttoned in some delicately obvious area. Without doubt, they can be a little different.

It stands to reason then that the family clown or entertainer is likely to be the last born. Nobody told me that—I just naturally assumed the role. I was the Dennis the Menace type. What I wanted was attention. That was my thing in life —getting people to laugh or point or comment. There were at least two good reasons for my thirst to achieve "stardom": a brother five years older who was 9.75 in everything and a sister eight years older who was a perfect 10.00. Ever since I could remember it seemed that I scored around 1.8 in comparison to their abilities and achievements.

But I was determined to get my share of the attention. As a five-year-old I went to a relative's wedding and became forever established in her memory book when it came time to throw the rice. Everyone was throwing rice but Kevin. I was throwing gravel.

No wonder, then, that when I turned eight and my cheerleader sister, Sally, invited me to become the "mascot" for the high school team I jumped at the chance. Hundreds of people came to those games and they would all be looking right at me! I loved every minute of it, even that embarrassing scene when I forgot the cheer and the crowd roared with laughter. In fact, at that moment, in the Williamsville High School gym, on a cold winter night in western New York, I made a life-changing decision. I decided to be an entertainer.

Yes, I know I came out a psychologist who is practicing family therapy every day with good results. I enjoy my chosen profession and get deep satisfaction from helping families, but my cherished avocation is making people laugh, and I do it whenever and wherever I can—in seminars, conventions, and during television and radio talk shows.

A typical characteristic of the last born is that he is more carefree and vivacious—a real "people person" who is usually popular in spite of (because of?) his clowning antics.

Get the family together for the big Thanksgiving or Christmas photo. Work tenaciously to maneuver everyone into place and to snap the shutter when everyone looks halfway sane and—whoops! Who's that over on the left with the crossed eyes trying to touch his nose with his tongue? Yes, it's last-born Buford (who in this picture may be twenty-six years old) doing his thing for a laugh.

Or maybe Buford is doing his thing for other reasons. There is another mainstream of qualities in most last borns. Besides being charming, outgoing, affectionate, and uncomplicated, they can also be rebellious, critical, temperamental, spoiled, impatient, and impetuous.

The "Clowns" Want to Be Taken Seriously

I can relate to this "dark side" of the last born. Without question, part of my motivation for being "clown prince" of the Leman family was that I wasn't born crown prince or princess. Sally and Jack had beaten me to it. It seemed to me they had all the talent, ability, and smarts. They had all the firepower and I was a dud.

These are typical feelings of the last-born child. Last borns carry the curse of not being taken very seriously, first by their families and then by the world. In fact, your typical last borns have a "burning desire to make an important contribution to the world."[1] From the time they are old enough to start figuring things out, last borns are acutely aware they are youngest, smallest, weakest, and least equipped to cope with life. After all, who can trust little Festus to set the table or pour the milk? He's just not quite "big enough" for that yet.

I like the description of last borns by Mopsy Strange Kennedy, a family therapist who on occasion writes for various magazines. Mopsy is a last born herself and that's no surprise. Only a last-born baby of the family is likely to grow up, get a degree, become a therapist, and still keep a handle that sounds like a nickname or pet label of some kind. And so Ms. Kennedy speaks from experience when she observes that the babies of the family "live, inevitably, in the potent shadow of those who were Born Before."[2]

I understand when Mopsy recalls how her early achievements (tying shoes, learning to read, telling time, etc.) were greeted with polite yawns and murmurings of, "Isn't that nice," or worse, "Horace, do you remember when Ralph learned to do that?" Ralph, of course, is the big brother born first. Last borns instinctively know and understand that their knowledge and ability carry far less weight than that of their older brothers and sisters. Not only do parents react with less spontaneous joy at the accomplishments of the last born; they may, in fact, impatiently wonder, *Why can't this kid catch on faster? His older brother had this down cold by the time he was two and a half.*

Part of the reason for this is that the parents get all "taught out" by the time the last born arrives. The tendency is to let the last born sort of shift for himself. It's not unusual for babies of the family to get most of their instruction from their brothers and sisters in many areas. The parents are just too pooped for any more pedagogy.

Obviously, receiving instructions from older brothers and sisters does not ensure that last borns are getting the facts of life (or anything else) very straight. Last borns are used to being put down. The older kids always laugh at the babies, who still grope blindly in fantasies like Santa Claus and the Tooth Fairy. It's no wonder the last born grows up with an "I'll show *them!*" attitude.

The Checkered Academic Career of Kevin the Clown

To "really show them I mattered" was one of my main motivations while growing up. Sally and Jack didn't make fun of me a lot. In fact, Sally became something of a second mother. But both of them certainly had it all over me in the achievement categories. I often describe the three of us in the same terminology used for reading groups at school. Sally, the $A+$ student, and Jack, the $B+$ student, were the "Bluebirds" of the family. I took one look at all this and decided to become the "Crow." Reading bored me and studying anything was the last thing I wanted to do—and I usually did it last, or not at all.

But I wanted—and desperately needed—attention and I got it by clowning, teasing, and showing off. I wasn't your classic juvenile delinquent. In fact, I could be quite charming (which probably saved my life a few times when I went too far with big brother, Jack).

Another thing you will read on the characteristic charts for last borns is that they are suckers for praise and encouragement. A little pat on the head, a slap on the back, and a "Go get 'em— we're counting on you" is enough to keep a last born going for hours, if not weeks.[3]

That was certainly the case when I was the mascot for the high school team. One of my most legendary feats involved a sneak attack on another school's mascot. Amherst Central High School was our mortal enemy in athletics, and their cheerleading squad included two guys who dressed up in a tiger suit and danced around on the sidelines during the basketball and football games. One night, as I watched from our side of the gym, a fantasy formed. What if I could sneak up on the tiger, yank off its tail, and run as fast as my eight-year-old legs could carry me back to our bench before anyone could stop me? Well, I did just that and made the high school paper with the banner headlines: "Demon Leman Defeats Amherst Tiger in Halftime Bout." With that kind of clipping, a last born barely needs food. He's living on praise.

But it's hard for a leopard (or a billy goat) to change its spots. Once I started getting all that reinforcement as a kid, I went on to develop clowning into a fine art. By the time I hit (literally) high school I was a master of sorts at getting laughs while driving teachers crazy.

I did all the dumb tricks: crawling out of class on my hands and knees, setting wastebaskets on fire, getting everyone in school to bring alarm clocks set for 2:00 P.M. and put them in their lockers. Today principals and teachers would shake their heads and go back to worrying about the newest dope pusher seen on campus. But twenty-five years ago those kinds of capers were a big deal and they got me big laughs. It got so the other kids would come into a class on the first day of the term, see me, and start nudging each other and smiling. Yes, this class was going to be a blast. Leman was in it!

When some birth order charts talk about a last born's charm they mention that he or she can be "a joy to have in a group or a class." Not for my teachers, I wasn't. As a high school senior I took a course called Consumer Math, a fancy term for bonehead arithmetic. They stuck me in there because it was the last term of the year and they didn't know what else to do with me.

The first six weeks I got a *C* and the second six weeks I pulled a *D*. During the third six weeks I was getting an *F* and was thrown out, but not before I had driven the teacher out as well. And I didn't just drive her out of class; I drove her out of teaching. She quit and didn't come back!

The poor woman just didn't know how to handle powerful attention getters like Leman. She thought I was out to get her. Not really—I was out to get laughs, admiration from my schoolmates, and the limelight. Very few of my teachers understood this, but one exception was an English instructor who kept me in line quite easily. He was so direct and businesslike that I knew my clowning would never work. As far as he was concerned, it was "shape up or you're out of here!" I shaped up. How can you get attention if you're not even there?

That instructor probably never heard the

term, but he was an expert in Reality Discipline, which is what I really wanted all the time, even more than the laughs and the attention. Last borns especially want and need Reality Discipline, which deals directly and swiftly with the student's problem and demands that he be accountable for his actions. We'll be looking more closely at Reality Discipline in Part Five, which will cover parenting.

I should have been a much better student—I had the ability—but the schools I grew up in did not hold me accountable. They just pushed me through. They wanted to get rid of guys like Leman—and the sooner the better. Very few of my teachers saw through my last-born charade. I have mentioned the no-nonsense English instructor. There was also a math teacher who wasn't fooled. As I came down to my last semester in high school she pulled me aside, looked me in the eye, and asked, "Kevin, when are you going to stop playing your game?"[4]

"What game is that, Teach?" I asked. (Yes, I actually did call her "Teach." After all, this was 1961 and we were "cool.")

"The game that you play the best," she smiled. "Being the worst!"

I laughed and tried to act as if I didn't care, but she had me. Her words began to turn my life around and they are still with me today. Recently, I visited with my math teacher and thanked her again for sounding the challenge that woke me up. She smiled and said, "Oh, I did very little, Kevin. You did it yourself. You were a challenge all right, but I knew what you could do if you wanted to!"

What a beautiful, unselfish lady. And rather modest, too. She didn't even mention that she tutored me at her home during those final weeks when I was making a last desperate gasp to graduate!

When my math teacher "blew my cover," so to speak, I went to the high school counselor and said, "I've been doing some heavy thinking and I want to go to college."

The counselor looked up at me over the top of his glasses and without hesitation replied, "Leman, with your record, I couldn't get you admitted to reform school."[5]

His response was a bit discouraging, but I could sort of understand where he was coming from. I was ranked fourth in my class—fourth from the bottom—going into my final semester.

"Okay, I'll show you," I muttered. "I'll get into college on my own!"

And I tried, yes, I really tried—160 schools in all. You could easily say I worked harder trying to get into college than I did to get out of high school.

In those days there weren't community colleges on every corner, with an open-door policy for anyone who was at least semiliterate. You either went on to school or you went to work. I had a real aversion to the latter, so I chose school—*any* school. It was pretty discouraging when every one of them turned me down, even our church denomination's college, North Park College in Chicago, Illinois.

But I wouldn't give up. I kept writing back to North Park and called in reinforcements to bombard the school with their letters, too. My brother, Jack, who had attended North Park for two years and later graduated from another college, sent a letter extolling my change of heart and determination to make it in college if given a chance. I also persuaded my pastor to write; I even sent in Scripture texts on the virtues of forgiving a wrongdoer seventy times seven![6]

Nine days before the semester started, North Park relented and let me in on probation with the understanding that I carry a twelve-unit load. During the first year the "fear factor" (fear of having to go to work) kept me going. Despite woefully weak preparation in high school, I eked out a *C* average. But then I ran out of gas. I guess I thought I didn't have anything left to prove. In my sophomore year I fell behind, and started failing fast.

I also failed in areas other than academic. Reverting to my high school habits, I sought attention by teaming with my roommate to rip off the ice-cream conscience fund (established because of a faulty machine which dispensed free ice cream) and buy pizza for our entire floor. We saw our crime as more of a prank than anything else. In fact, we made sure we told everyone we had done it. How can you get attention if you don't advertise?

Two days later I attracted the kind of attention I didn't want. The dean called me in and asked if I knew anything about the theft of the conscience money. In true last-born fashion I manipulated things a bit and said, "Yes, sir, I have heard that unfortunately some inconsiderate person has stolen the conscience box."

Well, the dean knew I was withholding evidence (i.e., lying through my teeth) and he had no choice. He suggested that I had had a hard year and I needed a rest—permanently—from North Park. I thought about his offer and it seemed like an appropriate time to leave. Spring weather is always nasty in Chicago. My parents had just moved to Tucson, Arizona, where it was nice and warm. I was failing my courses and the dean had completely failed to see any humor in the conscience-fund caper.

And so I left school and went home to Tucson, where I got a job as a janitor. It was while I was cleaning urinals that the realities of life sort of hit Baby Kevin right in the eye. Yes, I had a year of college behind me and I knew I could do it if I wanted to. But here I was, a janitor making $195 a month full time.

After cleaning a few more toilets I decided that really wasn't what I wanted to do in life. I

143

enrolled in a night course at the University of Arizona and promptly flunked it.

Maybe I will have to wind up a janitor after all, I was thinking one day as I emptied the trash at the men's rest room door, when I looked up and around the corner of the hallway came my wife. Of course, she wasn't my wife yet, but she was a very beautiful nurse's aide who was working in the building.

My first words were, "How would you like to go to the New York World's Fair with me?"

She laughed and said, "I don't think so."

"Well," I said. "How about lunch, maybe?"

Sande didn't quite know what to make of this weird fellow who was going around the building emptying trash, but being a nurse's aide she thought I might need help, so she agreed to a lunch date. We wound up at McDonald's, where we split a twenty-cent cheeseburger.

We kept dating and soon we were going steady. Sande could tell that I was searching for something in life and she shared her personal faith in God with me. It was through Sande that I made some spiritual commitments that at last turned me in the direction my math teacher had pointed way back in high school. I took another course at the University of Arizona, similar to the one I had flunked, and I passed with a solid *A,* highest grade in the class of six hundred.

From there I went on to get my undergraduate degree in psychology, followed by master's and doctorate degrees. And I was on the dean's list most of the way through. A lot of things motivated me: memories of my English and math teachers, memories of getting a start at North Park and blowing it with stupid pranks, meeting Sande and getting my life squared away by finding a real faith in God.

But there was also a remark made by Sande's supervisor in her nursing ward. This middle-aged lady pulled Sande aside one day and said, "Don't associate with that janitor—he'll never amount to anything." A comment like that is enough to spur any last born on to greater heights.

Last Borns: Perceptive People Persons

Long before now you've noticed I'm not bashful about using illustrations from my own family, not to mention my own life. But I turned this chapter into a miniautobiography for a reason. My antics as a kid and on up through high school are a classic demonstration of many typical last-born traits that can go to seed and become destructive. Frankly, before my math teacher nailed me that day in the hallway between classes, I was headed for real disaster. She made me realize that getting attention was not enough. Somehow it registered in my teenage brain that "the limelight is fun, Leman, but what do you do for an encore?" And that drove me on to a goal I had never even thought about—college degree.

I like to describe myself as one of the few certified psychologists I know who went through college and postgraduate work—thirteen years in all—without the benefit of a high school education. I literally did not learn much of anything in high school, a fact that hardly makes me proud.

Every summer I return for a week to a camp operated by our church denomination to speak to teenagers. I tell them my story and emphasize that my behavior as a youth is hardly the kind they want to imitate. In fact, I let them know, just as my math teacher let me know, that being best at being worst is a stupid game for anyone to play.

It's important, however, to realize that when I changed directions I didn't totally change my last-born nature. I had always been people oriented and I wound up in a very people-centered profession—counseling and teaching. Studies show that babies of the family gravitate toward vocations that are people oriented, while first borns and only children tend to like jobs involving the handling of data, materials, or other "things."

Car Salesmen Are Often Last Borns

Have you ever walked onto a used car lot to be greeted by a guy with a big smile, white shoes, matching white belt, dark blue pants, light blue shirt, and dark blue polka-dot tie? Maybe he wasn't dressed quite that flashy, but his first words probably were, *"Well,* what would it take to put *you* in *that* car today?"

If you've ever had such an encounter it's likely you were dealing with the baby of the family. You have to be careful with these guys— they'll sell you your own house and throw in a paint job by the owner to boot!

I jest a bit, but essentially it's true. Your good salespeople are often last borns. I do some consulting with businesses and one of my favorite stops is a car dealership. I was visiting a local car agency one day and started talking casually with one of the salesmen about birth order. It turned out he was a last born and so was just about every salesman in the agency! And what about the manager? I went with the odds and guessed he was a first born. Right again. First borns often wind up in positions of leadership. This manager was an excellent salesman in his own right, but as a first born he had risen to what he really wanted to do; cross the *t*s, dot the *i*s, and enter those nice black numbers on the bottom line.

Interestingly enough, this first-born manager was having trouble with some of his last-born salesmen. They just weren't attending to details such as filling in reports on time, etc., etc. Not surprisingly, his superstar salesman was a last born and was in the most hot water with the manager. I sat down with the manager for a cup of coffee and had him consider: "What do you really want this guy to do—sell or do paperwork?"

The manager's answer boiled down to "both."

I recommended to the manager that he stop trying to turn a baby of the family into a perfectionist. Why not alleviate the problem by arranging to have one of the secretaries or clerks do the paperwork and turn his salespeople loose to do what they do best—sell!

The manager took my advice and assigned a clerk to fill in the salesman's paperwork for him. Naturally enough, his sales went higher than ever, and it meant more money for the dealership.

Last Borns Live With Ambivalence

In my research on birth order, I often run across the idea that growing up the youngest can turn you into a bundle of uncertain ambivalence. Last borns are on a seesaw of emotions and experiences that they find hard to explain or understand.[7] My own life as the last born bears this out. We babies of the family can be charming and endearing one minute, rebellious and hard to deal with the next. We can turn from powerhouses of energy into basket cases who feel helpless. We can feel on top of the world on Monday and at the bottom of the pile on Tuesday.

I'm not sure about the exact reasons for this ambivalent streak that we babies of the family carry through life, but here are a few clues. Last borns are treated with ambivalence—coddled, cuddled, and spoiled one minute, put down and made fun of the next. In self-defense we babies of the family grow up with an independent cockiness that helps cover all our self-doubt and confusion. We say to ourselves, "They wrote me off when I was little. They wouldn't let me play. They chose me last. They didn't take me seriously. *I'll show them!*"

Beneath our independent veneer is that inner rebel who got away with murder. We last borns are impetuous and brash. We go ahead and *do it* and worry about repercussions later. We vow that we will get attention, we will make our mark. We will show our older brothers and sisters, our parents, and the world that we are to be reckoned with.

I'm sure that's what drove me to be such a little demon while growing up. I couldn't compete with a 10.00 sister and a 9.75 brother, but I could get their attention by driving them crazy. I especially loved teasing Sally, the first-born perfectionist, who made a career of putting all her ducks in a row and marching them through life in flawless formation. Besides, teasing Sally was safer. She couldn't punch as hard as Jack!

Possibly my finest hour came when Sally got married. She was in her early twenties and I was a teenager. Sally couldn't figure out how to involve me in her wedding. She couldn't trust me to be an usher—who knows what I would pull right in the middle of the ceremony? So, she assigned me to take care of the guest book.

The night before her wedding, we all attended the traditional rehearsal dinner at a fashionable downtown hotel. Even I showed up dressed to kill, in a suit and tie. As custom would have it, Sally gave everyone involved in the wedding a little gift. I opened mine and discovered a bright plaid pair of Bermuda shorts. Another fantasy formed and Leman the demon could not resist. I slipped out and did a quick Clark Kent change in a nearby rest room. Moments later, I reappeared in the swank hotel dining room attired in suit coat, tie—and the shorts!

Sally's face turned bright red as her perfect evening dissolved into guffaws by the guests and menacing looks from the maître d'. But I was happy. Once again I was the center of attention. I would pay the price later when I faced Mom and Dad at home, but it was worth it. Once again I had struck a blow for all the last borns who have ever vowed, "I'll show them!"

Tips for Last Borns
Making Your Birth Order Work for You

If you are a baby of the family, some of the following suggestions can help you cope with life today as an employee, spouse, parent, and friend.

1. Accept responsibility for yourself. Maybe for the first time you should stop passing the buck. You're not a little kid anymore, so why continue acting like it? As those girls back in seventh grade used to say, "Grow up!"

2. Many last borns are "messies." Learn to pick up after yourself. Your spouse will rise up to call you blessed and your mother may say, "I never thought I'd see the day. . . ."

3. Take stock of where you are right now in your present job. Are you working with people? You are quite likely a people person, and that's where you will find the most opportunity and satisfaction. Perhaps you should consider changing your line of work, even if it means a temporary cut in pay. Sales work is a strong possibility, but so is any job that requires interaction with people. You might also consider a managerial

slot, *as long as you feel you can keep things organized and on schedule.*

4. While last borns are usually people persons, ironically they struggle with self-centeredness. Offer to help others, then follow through and quietly do it without fanfare. Helping others —sharing your money, time, and energy—is a great cure for self-centeredness.

5. Beware of being too independent. Work on admitting your faults. Don't blame others for your situation when you know you're the one who really caused it.

6. Always be aware of your gift to be funny, charming, and persuasive. Use it correctly and you will be an asset in any situation. Beware, however, of being a carrot seeker, always working for that pat on the head, and always asking, "What's in it for me?"

7. If you love the limelight, be advised that other people like a little of it now and then, too. When talking with others, always concentrate on asking them about their plans, their feelings, and what they think.

8. Before marriage, try dating first borns. You may find them the most compatible. After marriage, to any birth order, remember that your wife is not your mommy, you husband is not your daddy. (For more on the best birth order combinations in marriage, see chapter 9.)

Part Four

Birth Order and Marriage: Some Better, Some Worse

There is no relationship where birth order has a more profound impact than marriage. Some combinations make excellent matches, others can lead to mayhem. The next two chapters deal with . . .

- why two first borns can end up fighting
- why two perfectionists seldom have a perfect marriage
- the secret of having a less-than-perfect—and happier—marriage
- why two middle children may not negotiate happily ever after
- why quiet, pleasing wives can drive some husbands away

- how two last borns can let the good times roll too far
- why a first-born wife and a last-born husband are usually so compatible
- how favorite "life lines" can ruin marriages, including:
  "I only count when I'm perfect."
  "I only count when I avoid conflict."
  "I only count when I'm noticed."
  "I only count when I'm in control."
- how to make any marriage work better

Chapter Eight

Birth Order Marriages Aren't Made in Heaven

"It's a marriage made in heaven."

You may have heard this comment on occasion. Maybe you made that comment yourself about your own marriage or at the wedding of two beautiful people who looked as if they couldn't miss the train bound for that fabled little hamlet called Happiness Everafter.

Before I started doing psychological counseling of couples and families, I used to think that marriages could be made in heaven. Now I know they are made on earth and my first question of any couple who comes for marital counseling is, "What is your birth order?"

The answer I get most often is, "I'm a first born and so is he," or, "I'm an only child and so is she."

This is not to say I don't counsel couples who are middle children or last borns, but over the years, as I have counseled hundreds of couples, the most competitive, most volatile, and most discouraged are combinations where both spouses are first borns or, worse, both are only children.

Like mountain sheep these couples seem to naturally butt heads. Their relationship is the opposite of the true concept of marriage: pulling together, sharing, melting into the unity of one. Many of the first-born or only-child couples I see are "one" only in the sense that they have locked horns over something and neither one will back off.

And what do they disagree about? Everything. First borns and only children are by nature perfectionistic flaw finders and nit-pickers. There's a country song that goes, "You want things your way and I want them mine." How true it is!

I recall one couple I threw out of my office because I got sick and tired of hearing them fight. Every time they came to see me, they spent the first ten or twenty minutes fighting. In fact, they started fighting in the waiting room and just continued when they came into my office. After several sessions of playing referee, I decided there would be no more fighting on company time.

"No charge for today," I said. "I'm sick and tired of listening to you two run each other down. You go home and think it over. When you're both ready to take a run at making a marriage, come see me again."

Admittedly, I used some rather harsh tactics, but I felt I had no choice. Over the years, I have only done this kind of thing approximately half a dozen times. Interestingly enough, it usually gets great results.

In this case, I began thinking I had probably blown it. I didn't hear from the couple for about a month. Just about the time I began thinking they enjoyed fighting too much to stop, they called for an appointment. They came, they didn't fight (at least in my presence), and eventually we got someplace in improving their marriage.

But the key that unlocked their horns, so to speak, was the decision to quit bumping heads. Couples just cannot continue to run each other down and expect their marriage to survive. It's like taking a chisel to the foundation of a huge building. One blow doesn't do much—it just chips off a little concrete. But use that chisel long enough and hard enough, and sooner or later the whole place comes down. And that's what I see couples doing—especially the first-born and only-child combinations. Their chisels are their tongues and they just keep chipping away.

I ask them, "How did all this start?" Their answer often involves "the little things"—it's the little things that drive first born nuts: clothes left in a heap, the unbalanced checkbook, the unentered check that unbalanced the checkbook in the first place. . . .

The major problem is perfectionism. They're both perfectionists in their own way, but each can do very "unperfect" things to the other and it's like striking a match around gasoline. Husbands who are letter perfect down at the office leave the bathroom and bedroom a mess. A favorite line I hear from the wife is, "Does he think I'm his mother?" Or, "Does he think I'm the maid?"

I might add that the "Do you think I'm your mother?" syndrome is not limited to first-born or only-child couples. It happens with other birth orders, too.

If I hope to make any progress with any couple, I must get them thinking about what they're doing to each other.

"Who's winning this marriage?" I ask. "With all the lambasting you're doing on one another, who is coming out on top?"

They usually look at each other and then back to me and one of them says, "Well, uh, nobody does. . . ."

"Exactly," I say, and then we work on the problem. The first problem is often quite simple. They married within their own birth order. I have already mentioned how volatile a marriage of two first borns or two only children can be. I see more of the discouraged-fast-becoming-destructive perfectionists than anybody else. But a marriage between two middle children can be destructive, too; so can a match with two babies.

The first principle (not a rule) for a riskier kind of marriage is this: Marry someone in your own birth order. If you want better odds for a happier marriage, marry out of your birth order. We'll discuss that later in this chapter, but right now let's take a look at some examples of couples who married within their own birth orders and see what happened.

The Perfectionists With a Sex Problem

Shirley, an attractive thirty-eight-year-old blonde, and George, a forty-one-year-old engineer, both first borns, came to see me with what George called "Shirley's sex problem." The oldest of four children, Shirley grew up in a family with an extremely domineering father, whom she described as "intelligent and explosive." According to Shirley, her dad had always tried to "run my life." And while still in her teens, she vowed she would "never marry anyone like Dad."

Of course, Shirley went out and married someone just like Dad and then some. I'm often asked just why people do this. It's impossible to know all the reasons for anyone's particular behavior, but we can make some good guesses. One way to explain Shirley is that as a rule the parent of the opposite sex has the most influence on us. In Shirley's case her domineering, critical father had made his mark. Despite all her vows to "never marry anyone like him," she had an even deeper drive she wasn't aware of that was saying, "I could never satisfy Dad, so I'll find a man just like him and please him. I'll win yet!"

But Shirley's first-born perfectionism doomed her to failure. With Shirley's approach to sex it's no wonder she developed a problem. For her sex was like everything else in her life—a carefully regimented performance. Intercourse for Shirley and George was done with little deviation in technique, position, lighting (none), etc. Shirley was a demanding person and the one she demanded the most from was herself.

George was also demanding. He wanted sex every day. The result of this combination of demands and drives was that Shirley was uptight, unable to enjoy intercourse, and growing more unresponsive to George who, a perfectionist in his own right, was constantly nit-picking her to death, particularly about sex.

The nit-picking, of course, just made Shirley all the more uptight and resentful. George was simply reminding his wife of how domineering her father had been.

The situation looked pretty bleak when Shirley and George began counseling. The one ray of hope was that they both wanted to save the marriage. Whenever I get counselees like these,

I am greatly encouraged. We are living in a day of "If it doesn't work out, chuck him [or her] and try someone else." But when I take any marriage counseling case, my goal is to save that marriage. My approach is simple and basic: If a couple has stood before God and man to say, "I do, for better or for worse," that couple should try everything possible to stay together.

The whole situation was a classic case of two first-born perfectionists locking horns and banging heads with no relief in sight. Our first step toward unlocking their horns was to suggest a less rigid and demanding schedule regarding sex. It wasn't too hard to sell them on this. Because of all the tension, they had already dropped down to "only" four times a week.

I gave them several assignments on how to relax and enjoy each other while they made sex a celebration instead of an ordeal. They made good progress as a couple and I also gave Shirley several assignments of her own that she carried out very well.

Assignment number one for Shirley was to "admit your perfectionist tendencies." One of the ways people can cope with their drive toward perfectionism is to admit, "I'm a perfectionist and I have to deal with this." This simple exercise starts making them much more aware of the demands they are placing on themselves, as well as on others.

Another assignment for Shirley was to "watch

those expectations." I wanted her to give herself fewer and smaller assignments, to take smaller bites in life. By not expecting so much from herself and from others, she would find it easier to forgive herself when she goofed or "blew it." And if she had to go to someone else to ask forgiveness, so much the better. She did start doing this in small ways with George, much to his amazement and pleasure.

A third assignment for Shirley was to "learn to say no." She had to start saying no to things she didn't want to do. At church, for example, she was known as "one who could always be counted on to help." Naturally, she always wound up doing double duty and carrying the load for herself as well as for several other people.

With some hard work on Shirley's part, she began to say no to requests. She began giving herself some space. She began ending the tyranny of the "to do" lists that she literally taped on the steering wheel of her car to constantly remind her of the next errand or appointment. She planned less during the day and was able to see herself "getting more things accomplished," rather than finishing each day irritated and frustrated because she had not "gotten everything done."

Just as predictably, the relationship between Shirley and George improved radically, particularly in bed. They started having sex less and enjoying it more! Something else Shirley had to deal with was her image of George as a very dominating husband. Rather than play a passive role to George, I encouraged her to take a certain amount of initiative when it came to sex. I suggested things like "kidnapping" her husband from work, having a motel room reserved, or getting out of town to a nearby resort for an overnight, taking time for a picnic lunch in the middle of a workday, etc.

Perfectionist that she was, she really threw herself into her new assignments with enthusiasm. I remember the delight with which she told me of the time she picked up George after work for an evening that included time in a hot tub, picnic supper, and a motel for the evening. She had made the reservations, arranged for Grandma to stay with the kids, etc.

While Shirley and George had problems, it was Shirley who was the key to getting this marriage back on the right track. As soon as she started dealing positively with her perfectionism, she was able to rearrange priorities. As she started controlling her own expectations and goal setting, the scene changed. By marrying a man much like her father—domineering and critical—she had set herself up for failure. It was like a train that had been roaring full speed toward a washed-out bridge. But Shirley stopped the train, threw a switch, and got herself and

George on a track that led to safety and happiness.

Sylvia Plus Mark Equaled No Communication

Another birth order marriage that can run into lots of trouble is that of two middle children. As we saw in chapter 6, the middle child shoots off in his own direction, depending on the strengths and weaknesses of the first born ahead of him. The middle child can go a lot of directions, but one basic characteristic most middle children develop is the ability to mediate, negotiate, and compromise. (See page 122.) This sounds like a wonderful skill to carry into marriage, but ironically what often happens with two middle children is a tendency to desire peace at any price. They become avoiders—of their problems and eventually each other. Middle children prefer the oceans of life to be smooth. They don't want to make waves and the result can be a "quiet surface," but underneath all kinds of storms are brewing because they are not communicating.

Such was the case with Sylvia, a thirty-two-year-old quiet brunette and third-born daughter in a family of five children. With two sisters above her and two boys below her, Sylvia got lost in the middle during childhood and teenage years. She grew up shy, passive, and definitely an avoider of conflict, who tried to please her parents by taking over a lot of the care of her two younger brothers while her mother worked.

Mark was twenty-nine, the second of three children. His older brother had always been the best at everything, and his baby sister got the typical "baby princess" treatment that often left Mark feeling as if he hadn't gotten a fair shake.

Mark went outside the family early to find his own friends and social life, another classic mark of the middle child (see chapter 6). One of those friends was Sylvia, his high school sweetheart, whom he married soon after graduation. After eight years of marriage, Sylvia and Mark had two children, seven and four years of age.

Sylvia arranged for the counseling, acting on the urging of one of her older sisters, who was tired of hearing her complain of feeling trapped with little children and unable to communicate with her husband. Sylvia was also worried about another woman because during the last few months Mark had been insisting he had to work longer hours at his job.

I talked separately with Sylvia, then Mark. It turned out there was no other woman. It seemed one woman was all Mark could handle, especially when she tried to "run me all the time." Sylvia was still operating with Mark the way she had with her two younger brothers. She kept telling him what to do and Mark resented it, even when it came from a sweet, shy girl like his wife. Sylvia was baffled, of course, and could not understand why Mark was spending so much time at work. Her answer was another woman. His answer was to stay away from feeling uncomfortable with the woman he already had. As a middle child, Mark didn't want to make waves. He wanted to avoid conflict whenever he could, so the simplest solution was, "Sorry, I have to work late tonight."

Sylvia, on the other hand, didn't know how to approach Mark and could only guess as to what was going on. Communication was at zero when Sylvia came to me for help. Sylvia and Mark made good progress when they committed themselves to spending time talking together, after the kids were in bed and they could concentrate on each other. Having Mark share his feelings really helped Sylvia because his silence and secretive devotion to work had bothered her a great deal. Mark learned he could tell Sylvia how he felt and she would not reject him.

While Sylvia appreciated the talks with Mark, she admitted it was difficult to verbally form her thoughts. I suggested that she supplement the talks by writing Mark positive little notes now and then. For example, Mark had to travel for his company every once in a while and Sylvia began slipping little notes and cards into his suitcase. Finding those little love notes and brief bits of encouragement in between his shirts, when he was unpacking in the motel, made the trips much easier for Mark.

I often advise spouses—especially wives—to write notes and send cards. After all, what does it really cost? A card might be a dollar and take a few minutes of time, but the result can be worth so very much to the marriage.

Another plus that came out of the new effort to communicate was that Sylvia felt less trapped as the mother of two small children while her husband had his outlet—his job. Mark learned to come home and say, "What can I do to help?" Sylvia was thrilled, and as Mark was willing to be more helpful around the house, she learned to back off on her "motherly little ways of telling him what to do."

As middle children, Sylvia and Mark were really good candidates for marriage. The irony in their situation, however, is what faces any couple when both of them are middle born. If they do not communicate, it is because their urge to avoid conflict and make the oceans of life smoother wins out over their natural tendency to be mediators and negotiators. It sounds like a paradox, but that's how relationships often flounder.

Peter and Mary: Born Last, First in Debt

Marrying your own birth order is often not a good idea for the babies in the family, either. On the positive side, two last borns might have a ball during their courtship, because they both have a fun-loving, go-for-broke nature. But going for broke is not much fun when you're married, and unless one spouse can take responsibility for not letting the good times roll too far or too fast, two last borns can be headed for money troubles.

By the time they came to see me, Peter and Mary, both last borns in their families, were in serious difficulties with the bank and several other creditors. They were in their early thirties and had no children. Pete had a good income, but they were hopelessly in debt. Every credit card balance was well over the maximum, several department store bills were overdue, and their car and ski boat were about to be repossessed. The only reason they weren't in trouble on a house payment was that they were renting an apartment. And the only reason they weren't behind in their rent was a no-nonsense landlord who threatened immediate eviction proceedings if the rent was even one day past the ten-day "grace" period.

All of this fiscal chaos led, of course, to marital warfare. Neither Pete nor Mary had been particularly overindulged as children, but when they got out on their married own they decided to live by the pleasure principle. If they saw something they wanted, they bought (that is, *charged*) it. They blamed each other for their overindulgence; ironically enough, both were also overweight. There was no control anywhere in sight.

My first step with Peter and Mary was putting them in touch with a financial counselor. He forced them to go on a budget. They had to turn over all their assets and give up all their credit and charge account cards. Then the counselor wrote to every creditor and arranged for payment of acceptable minimum amounts on each account until everything could be paid off. Peter brought the cards in for me to see—all cut in small pieces. This sounds like a childish way to treat two adults, but it was their only hope. Last borns, as a rule, are the last people who can live on a tight budget. As a last born myself, I understand that perfectly. I never could operate on a tight budget; I leave it to my first-born wife, Sande, to keep us out of debt.

As soon as Mary and Peter restored a little order in their financial picture, they were able to work on their marriage. The debts and pressures from their creditors had been pulling them apart. With the pressure off, they were able to see that they had to pull together instead of in opposite directions. This pulling together included having one checking account, not two.

While living with their money mess, they had used separate checking accounts and, of course, each had bounced checks without telling the other.

Mary and Peter saw me only a few times. Their real problem was money, not their marriage. They loved each other and were committed to staying together. Once they committed themselves to not buying anything on credit for at least two years, and to sell a couple of their toys, like the ski boat, they were well on their way to stability.

Peter and Mary were typical examples of how lack of order and stability are often weak links in the makeup of last borns. As we saw in chapter 7, the last-born child grows up spoiled, overindulged, coddled, and cuddled. This hardly helps him get basic training for running a budget. On the other side of the coin, last borns are often treated as if they don't know quite enough, are always behind, too young, too small, too weak, too dumb. Last borns often develop an attitude that says, "Who cares anyway? You might as well have a little fun while it's there." Once Peter and Mary realized they could control their spending and still have fun, they enjoyed life with each other a whole lot more.

Which Birth Orders Make the Best Matches?

One of the leading birth order researchers in the field is Walter Toman, whose book *Family Constellation* is considered a classic study of more than three thousand families.[1] In discussing basic types of sibling positions, Toman lists what he believes are the best combinations for marriage among birth orders. Good matches, according to Toman, include:

The youngest brother of sisters with the oldest sister of brothers.
The youngest sister of brothers with the oldest brother of brothers.

My counseling experience proves Toman is right. The best match for a last born is obviously a first born—someone who is conscientious and a little more confident about having life together and keeping it that way. By the same token, the fun-loving nature of the last born can help loosen up the first born's typically overserious, conscientious approach to life. Possibly the best match one can find is the first-born female and the last-born male. First-born females are often mothering types and last-born males often need mothering.

I was fortunate enough to be the last-born brother of oldest sister, Sally, who mothered me quite a bit and taught little Kevin a lot about "What is a woman?"

I think most marriage counselors would agree that men do not understand women very well. *Any* extra learning a boy can get while growing up is going to help him later when he has a family of his own. In my case, however, I needed some postgraduate work, and Sande was happy to oblige.

How Mama Bear Reformed Cubby Bear

While it's a good rule of thumb to say that any combination of first born and last born has a better chance for happiness, it *does not* follow that success comes automatically. Good marriages are made, not born. Good marriages are made by two people who work at making them good by being considerate, caring, and mutually supportive.

When first-born Sande married last-born Kevin it was a classic match-up of the pleasing mama bear taking on the playful cub. And of course the cub took advantage of his new care giver. Sande soon learned that I liked only peas and corn, never, never lettuce, and I wasn't even too fond of *steak!*

And since I had always gotten away with taking off my clothes and letting them drop wherever I happened to be, I continued tossing socks, shirts, etc. on the floor and Sande went around picking them up.

This went on through the early years of our marriage. One day, while I was working on my doctor's degree, Sande heard me expostulating on the merits of Reality Discipline and holding children accountable for their actions.

The light dawned.

If holding children accountable for their actions is good, holding husbands accountable might even be better, Sande thought. She went into action.

I began catching on when I found my little piles of clothes where I had left them. Soon the entire apartment was covered with little piles. And then came the day when I could not open the door because it got stuck on a giant pile that she had shoved up against it to get it out of her way.

And so, Sande and I had the same kind of talk I now advise for a lot of couples who come to see me. We shared feelings. She said, "Look, I want to be your wife, not your mother. You learn to pick up your own clothes and put them where they belong. Also, I'm going to fix what I fix. I expect you to at least try different dishes. You owe that much to yourself and to our children—if you want to be the good role model you keep talking about."

Sande helped me grow up in other ways by introducing me to the pediatrician. In fact, she started allowing me to take Holly to the pedia-trician.

In short, Sande started expecting me to be a leader in our home and to take an active role in meeting the responsibilities. She even taught me that changing diapers was not off limits for a psy-chologist with a doctor's degree. *Parenthood isn't woman's work.*

And so I learned how to be Papa Bear instead of Cubby Bear. The moral of the story is that first borns should never let last-born spouses take advantage of them with their manipulative ways. And, of course, last borns should not be victimized by a first born who wants to do *too much* mothering or fathering.

Putting Your Marriage in Order

Whenever you think about which birth order can make the "best" marriage, you must always remember a key principle I keep repeating throughout this book:

> In matters of birth order, all general state-ments are indicators, not rules.

Because I say that in most cases a first-born/last-born marriage combination has a better chance for happiness, it does not follow that other combinations do not. For example, if you are married to someone in your own birth order, this is hardly an excuse to say, "Well, it's hopeless. I can see that John will never change and we're both doomed to divorce."

Many people marry in their birth order and have perfectly fine relationships. My own first-born sister, Sally, is an example. She married first-born Wes, a meticulous perfectionist who is a dentist. According to what we have said in this chapter, Sally and Wes should have picked each other apart by now, but such is not the case. They have built a great marriage around a common faith, a sense of balance, and plenty of hard work. And, they have three super kids to boot!

So, the good news is that birth order is never a final determinant of anything, but it is an indication of problems or tensions that you might discover—or create for yourself—as you go through life. What I try to do when I counsel any couple is to show them that in order for them to make a marriage work, they must work together. They must communicate and they must support and encourage, not pick and criticize. What they need to do is very basic. There is no great mystery to making a marriage work, but there is a great deal of difficulty. Knowing the characteristics of your birth order and knowing yourself better is one of the first steps to learning how to get along with your mate and building a happy life together.

Quiz for Every Married Couple

1. Do I nitpick? Do I find fault in what my mate wears, says, or does? How often?

2. Do I take the time to encourage my mate?

3. Do we talk things out? Have we set a time "just for us"?

4. When was the last time we took a weekend away from the children?

5. When was the last time I gave my mate a compliment?

6. When was the last time I gave my mate a special present for absolutely no particular reason except to say, "I love you"?

7. Speaking of "I love you," when was the last time I said those three little wonderful words to my mate?

8. What is the one thing I *know* my mate would love to have me do? Am I planning to do it this week?

9. Do we worship together? Or are we like too many couples who seem to have decided that God has joined the Edsel and other obsolete models?

10. Do I take the time to find out what my mate is really interested in? Do I take the time to understand the "ins and outs" of his or her favorite pastime or activity?

11. When was the last time I "kidnapped" my mate from the office (or maybe from the ironing board) and went away on an overnight?

12. When was the last time I came home early from work to take care of little Buford or Festus and let my mate go window shopping or run some errands?

13. When was the last time I said, "I am sorry. I was wrong. Will you forgive me?"

Chapter Nine

I Only Count When I . . .

How you complete that statement says a lot about you—and your marriage. When couples are having problems and have decided to "try the psychologist," one of the first things I look for is the life-style of each spouse. By "life-style" I don't mean how much money they make, where they live, or how many cars they drive. A better way to say it might be "style of life," which is a phrase Alfred Adler coined when talking about how people function psychologically to reach their goals. Adler believed that everyone develops a style of life while growing up. Several important influences are always present. Birth order automatically comes into play, along with foundation of sex roles, adjusting to circumstances and problems, and so on.

Adler taught that knowing a person's circumstances and his typical reflex actions toward circumstances told him nothing of what went on in that person's soul. But, wrote Adler, ". . . If I know the goal of a person, I know in a general way what will happen."[1] This goal determined what Adler called the person's "life line"—how that person described his perception of himself and what he was trying to do with his life.[2]

To keep things simple for our purposes, let's say our "style of life" is our perception of how we fit into our world. As we grow up through early childhood and gain certain perceptions of ourselves, we develop what Adler called "life lines" to go with our style of life. Adler's definition of *life line* can get quite technical, but simply speaking, I like to refer to life lines as the lines of talk we feed ourselves and learn to believe about ourselves.

The aggressive male is often tagged by the ladies as "a guy with a great line." Well, I believe we *all* have great lines and we use them on ourselves the most. These life lines all begin with, "I only count (am valuable or worthy) when I . . ." How we finish these lines is almost always directly connected to our birth order.

There are many life lines. Some of the more popular ones I often hear when I am counseling include:

"I only count when I'm perfect."
"I only count when I avoid conflict."
"I only count when I'm noticed."
"I only count when I'm in control."

Any of the above are excellent weapons for wrecking a marriage. Let's see why.

"I Only Count When I'm Perfect"

We learn these life lines very early. For example, a preschool teacher gives little Marilou a pair of scissors (rounded tips, of course) and a sheet of bright red construction paper. Marilou's assignment is to cut out a nice big circle. She labors away and is doing a fairly nice job when all of a sudden she crumples up the paper and throws her half-completed circle on the floor.

The teacher comes over and asks, "Marilou, what's wrong?"

"I can't do this!"

"I'll help you—here, let me—"

"No! I'm not going to do it. It's dumb!"

And teacher sighs and wonders, *What's gotten into Marilou?*

Well, let's give the teacher a few clues:

Marilou is a first-born child and her parents are both very competent people. What do you do when you are around very competent role models? You want to be like them. Just last week, Marilou made her own bed and did a very good job for a five-year-old. Mom came in to check it and said, "Oh, Marilou, honey, what a beautiful job you did." And then Mom proceeded to "straighten out a few wrinkles."

The message for Marilou? She didn't measure up. The bed wasn't "perfect."

No wonder that a less-than-perfect circle drives Marilou to distraction and mild insurrection at preschool. If she can't be perfect, she won't be anything at all!

And what does the story of Marilou at preschool have to do with marriage? A great deal. Let's jump ahead twenty or twenty-five years. Marilou is now married and like 50 percent of the wives today, she works outside the home. She arrives at the door, tired and hungry after a tough day on the job. Husband Burt got home first but he has forgotten to take the chicken out of the freezer and set the table. In addition, the sink is overflowing with dirty dishes and Burt is watching the sportscast on the six o'clock news.

This scene is enough to send any working wife up the wall, but when you add the fact of Marilou's perfectionism and wanting everything just so, you can expect real trouble. And that's just what she gives Burt, with a verbal barrage that makes him wonder what he ever saw in the six o'clock news anyway.

The trouble is, a few more of these perfectionistic pyrotechnics and Burt will be wondering what he ever saw in Marilou.

Marilou is trapped in a life-style that is built around the life line that says, "I only count when I'm perfect." Furthermore, people around her have to be perfect and when they aren't, she goes up like a space shuttle launch.

How do I counsel Marilou? Do I give her a lot of technical explanations about her mother and the danger of mild neuroses due to escapist tendencies? What I usually say is that if I've learned anything in almost twenty years of my own marriage, it's that life isn't perfect and no marriage is perfect. But when one or both mates is perfectionistic, that's when the trouble starts.

The perfectionist tries to enforce his or her standards on the spouse. This is where the cheap shots come in. One spouse tells the other, "You don't measure up," or "You're not good enough." What is happening is that one spouse is trying to change the other and it just doesn't work. Trying to change your mate takes its deadly toll on your marriage. You are wasting your breath. The only person you can change is yourself.

But it is hard to tell a perfectionist, "You can't change your mate." Perfectionists never give up, or they at least don't go down without a fight. I try to tell the perfectionist spouse that perfectionism isn't a bad trait, if you are a quality-control inspector on the assembly line and are paid to spot flaws from fifty yards. But perfectionism is deadly when you start spotting flaws from across the breakfast table.

Some other advice I try to give the perfectionist spouse includes the following:

1. *Avoid comparing yourself or your mate with other husbands or wives.* You are not some other husband or some other wife. You are you—you have a right to be yourself and so does your spouse.

2. *Ventilate feelings to yourself out loud.* Yes, I recommend talking to yourself. People who have a hard time talking to others can really do much better by talking to themselves and learning to articulate their feelings that way. Later, they can deal with communicating with the spouse.

3. *If perfection is your goal, you'll always feel a void in your life.* You'll never get there. It is a hopeless, fruitless quest. You must have the courage to accept yourself as you are—an imperfect person who is still learning, growing, and changing.

4. *Put your mate's feelings first—ahead of yours.* I know this is in contradiction to the psychology that seems to be in vogue in the 1980s, but I advise it anyway, because it works. Putting other people first—practicing the Golden Rule—is timeless wisdom that never goes out of style.

5. *Recognize that housework and office work will always be there, but will your mate—or your kids, who grow up so quickly?* Take time each week for a date with your spouse—in or out of the house. It doesn't have to be expensive, but what counts is that you have time to talk together about yourselves. Without this time for each other, your relationship can easily become empty and sterile. Commit yourselves to these special times, at least once a week, and stick with it even if the first few attempts don't go too well. It takes time

to learn to talk together, but the dividends are well worth it!

"I Only Count When I Avoid Conflict"

At the other end of the spectrum from the perfectionists are the people who seldom criticize. They aren't hung up on perfectionism. "Live and let live" is their model. They believe in peace at just about any price. Their life line reads, "I only count in life when I avoid conflict . . . when I don't make waves and the boat doesn't rock."

If you want to poison a marriage, this is another powerful life line to use. It is almost as effective as, "I only count when I'm perfect." Middle-born children are very susceptible to believing they only count when they avoid conflict because they've been negotiating and mediating all through life (see chapter 6). First borns who are the pleasing types are also frequent victims. The pleaser is the person who never offended Mom and Dad and now he or she surely doesn't want to offend his spouse, or the neighbors, or the pastor, or even the dog.

One principle I try to teach the avoiders of conflict and the pleasers is this: "Become expert at articulating your feelings in an acceptable way," with emphasis on "acceptable."

The pleasers and conflict avoiders stuff their

feelings deep inside and pay a terrible price physically and/or emotionally. The resentment builds and literally attacks the skeletal system and lining of the stomach in the form of ulcers, migraines, arthritis, etc. And it also oozes out to corrode the marriage relationship in the form of polite tension to poor or mundane sex life, from bickering to eventual blowups and knock-down, drag-out battles that usually mark the end of the marriage.

Recently I counseled a man in his second marriage who was a middle child, the classic easygoing, wouldn't-harm-a-fly type. He really wants to avoid conflict. So whom did he marry? An absolutely fascinating woman who seemed stimulating and interesting during the courtship. But once she walked down the aisle and said the vows, she turned into a badger.

An only child, this lady is in her first marriage and it is definitely a his-and-hers arrangement. Her life line is one we will look at a bit later: "I only count when I'm noticed." Like a lot of lonely onlies, she was given a great deal of attention as a child. She is used to being taken seriously. When her husband tried to avoid conflict, she read it as not taking her seriously enough, and that was when the fur would fly.

Why does a middle-born avoider of conflict marry an explosive woman like this? One explanation is that at a subconscious level he is motivated to team up with a spunky, abrasive person because those are the elements that are missing from his own personality. If you can't be a badger, the next best thing is to marry one, even though you pay for it down the line!

One of the major bones of contention in this marriage, which was less than a year old, was the husband's former wife and sixteen-year-old son. Anytime he would have any kind of communication with either the former wife or the son, his new bride would become incensed. The husband came to see me because his stomach was in knots. I tried to get him to tell me how he felt when his wife came unglued and he said, "I feel like running from her."

I asked if he could be more specific. "How do you really feel about what she says?"

"It makes me angry," he said. "It makes me feel as if she is trying to cut off my relationship with my sixteen-year-old son. I've had a relationship with him for sixteen years and I've known her a total of one year and eight months."

"Good point," I said. And then I talked with his wife and told her that one way to learn to love her husband would be to give him the freedom to have a relationship with his son. It turned out that her main concern was that he didn't discipline the boy enough! "He lets him do this and he lets him do that," she complained.

"Of course," I said. "He lets him do this and do that—do you know why? Because he wants to avoid conflict. He's being a permissive parent in order to steer clear of having to confront the boy."

It took several sessions to get the wife to understand her husband's lack of desire to do battle, verbal or otherwise. Her main problem was realizing that she had to accept her husband the way he was. She could not change him and the last way that she could get him to notice her was to rant and rave and carry on. This only drove him deeper into his shell.

I urged her to try another tack. Instead of discouraging her husband's relationship with his son, why not encourage it? The woman agreed and began inviting the boy over to the house. The happy result was that a great relationship developed between the sixteen-year-old and his stepmother. More important, the marriage rapidly improved when the wife gave the husband a little breathing room.

As this story demonstrates, avoiders of conflict often need help with communicating, or what I prefer to call "just plain speaking up" and letting each other know how they feel. Sometimes I'm challenged by people who think I'm suggesting that conflict is really a good thing. Churchgoers in particular tell me, "Dr. Leman, I don't get it. My pastor tells me, 'Happy are the peacemakers,' and you tell me, 'Miserable are the peacemakers.' What's going on here?"

Perhaps a better way to describe the conflict

avoider's life line is, "I only count when I make peace at any price." Don't misunderstand. I am not for war in a marriage. Making peace is a lot better, and usually a lot more fun. But there are those moments when one or both spouses must confront attitudes or behaviors that are damaging to the marriage. The trick is to make war on what is wrong, not on each other.

Peace at any price is no way to build the quality and oneness that every marriage needs. And ironically, when one partner avoids conflict by not saying anything, it actually creates more conflict, because nothing gets solved and the cause of the conflict continues to fester.

Other suggestions I have for couples who have a hard time confronting each other include these:

1. *Never forget that what* you *have to say and think is unique.* There's no one like you in the whole world, and the world needs your contribution.

2. *When you feel yourself shrinking from a social situation or even a conversation, push yourself to stay with it.* Force yourself to add your two cents. You'll be surprised to see that people will respond in a positive way. Who knows, they might even like what you have to say. How can you ever know if you don't try?

3. *Along that same line, if you find that you are putting yourself down before making a social contact, or trying something new, stop it immediately.* There

are already enough people in this mixed-up world who will be happy to step on you if you give them a chance. You don't need to join them.

4. *Do some heavy thinking about this one: When you are retiring, an avoider of any kind of confrontation or conflict, etc., you're not being humble or shy.* You don't deserve pity or sympathy. Actually, when you don't share your thoughts and your feelings with others, you are being selfish. Avoiding confrontation may seem like the easy way out, but sharing is a lot more constructive.

5. *Realize it's difficult to change.* You have spent most of your life following the path of least resistance. You can't expect to feel totally different overnight. Developing a new image will take patience and lots of adjustments—two steps forward, one step back is the name of the game.

"I Only Count When I'm Noticed"

Last borns often like this life line. They need to have fun, enjoy themselves, put others in their service, and manipulate. I shared part of my own last-born story in chapter 7, but I saved one little anecdote to illustrate what happens when you put a manipulative last-born husband together with a pleasing, gullible first-born wife.

Just before we were to be married, I told Sande there was a tradition in the Leman family that said the wife had to buy the marriage license. One of the strong traits in many first borns is a willingness to please other people, which comes, of course, from pleasing Mommy and Daddy, the main role models early in life. Unlike later-born children, the pleasing first born is not so likely to be worldly wise and alert to the wiles of those who would take advantage. In a word, my lovable wife is an easy mark.

So, it was not surprising that she thought it was wonderful when I asked her to fork over five dollars for a wedding license. I took the five-dollar bill from her, laid it on the marriage license clerk's desk, and said: "You've just started a tradition."

She just laughed. I laughed, too. We both knew I was trying to get through graduate school and was flat broke. She had the job, owned the car, and was our sole means of support. The whole thing was good for a laugh then, and we still chuckle about it today. At the time, we both got a harmless payoff for the life-styles we followed. I got noticed and had some fun; Sande got to play the pleasing role she enjoys so much.

But a life line such as "I only count when I'm noticed" can turn into a sour life-style in some cases. That's what happened to Butch and Stephanie, who came in for counseling after a marriage of only two years. Butch had caught Stephanie in lies on several occasions regarding her relationship to certain men. The last straw was Stephanie's weekend with one of the clerks at the store where she worked—a teenager four years her junior. As I got filled in on Stephanie's style of life, which she had developed as a child, it wasn't too surprising to learn that this precocious manipulator was the third and last born of three daughters. She had been spoiled as a young child, particularly by her father.

But the key piece of information was that Stephanie's parents had been divorced just about the time she turned ten. When Stephanie's dad moved out, she felt abandoned. Confused and hurt, she retreated into a shell as far as males were concerned.

Stephanie went through junior high and high school longing for some warm male input. When Butch came along right after she graduated from high school, she grabbed him. Butch was a good catch for Stephanie in many ways. A pleasing sort of middle child, he only wanted to make her happy. He came from a very stable home where there was lots of love and no divorce problems.

Butch filled in nicely as the daddy that Stephanie hadn't had for so long, but when you marry, you are supposed to be the husband or the wife, not the parent or the child. Butch made the mistake of giving Stephanie everything she wanted. That didn't keep her faithful. She paid him back by going out with other men—usually on one-night stands. And then she looked Butch right in the eye to tell him she had been faithful. Like many last borns, she was a great manipulator of people and was a master at putting the bits and pieces together in a way that sounded plausible and truthful.

Even while in counseling, Stephanie continued playing her promiscuous game. Psychologically she was in a double bind. First, she was hurting and resentful because her father had deserted her as she entered adolescence. Second, while she desperately wanted love from a male, she was afraid of it. Stephanie kept sending herself two messages: "I'm not worth a nice guy like Butch," and "I'll get back at my father any way I can."

Butch was caught in the middle and had to take it in the neck while his wife worked out her hostility toward her father. I see this a great deal. The husband winds up paying for the sins of the wife's father, and in other cases, the wife can pay for the sins of the husband's mother.

This story does not have a happy ending. No matter what we tried during counseling, it didn't help Stephanie. She was a compulsive liar and continued to try to destroy Butch with adulterous affairs. He finally bailed out and dissolved the marriage.

The "I only count when I'm noticed" life line is a bit deceptive because, after all, everyone likes to be noticed. No one enjoys it when a spouse, friend, boss, etc., pays no attention. What I am concerned about, however, is an *unhealthy* need for attention, the kind of need that drives a person to say, "I'll *make* you notice me. I'll get your attention one way or another."

On its extreme side, this kind of drive helps produce a Stephanie who, as a spoiled baby of the family, grew up to marry Butch and seek attention with adulterous one-night stands that destroyed their marriage. Ironically, Butch was giving her a great deal of attention, but in Stephanie's eyes it wasn't enough.

Granted, Stephanie's problem was an extreme one, and there were other psychological factors that played a part. But on its milder side, this "please notice me" life line can still eat away at a marriage. My advice includes the following points:

1. *The partner who needs all the attention is living selfishly, trying to outshine or outdo the other.*

2. *All these ploys to gain attention are what I call "carrot seeking." Last borns are particularly susceptible to carrot seeking because they want the payoff or limelight. But the trouble with carrot seeking is that you don't always grab your carrot. Sometimes you just don't get noticed.*

3. *To help carrot seekers become more mature, I suggest they do more giving and working behind the scenes in a deliberate effort to break their attention-seeking habits.*

"I Only Count When I'm in Control"

Another life line I see quite often in the people I counsel sounds like this: "I only count when I'm in control."

People who have to dominate and control do much better in "arm's length" relationships. They are often first borns or only children, but they can be of other birth orders as well. They are often the successful, achieving types—what I call the "Bluebirds" of life. But put them to a task requiring real intimacy with someone else— really opening up—and they are usually in trouble.

Controllers are the kind of people who are afraid to open up to their mates and tell them who they really are, what they're really like, and what they think about. Why are they afraid? If they had enough nerve, they would say, "If I tell you who I really am, you'll reject me." This is an exceptionally basic fear and almost all people struggle with it to some extent. Controllers really have a problem in this area.

In order to cover up this fear of intimacy, the controller dominates the other person in the relationship in several ways. A favorite approach is the hot temper. Such was the case with Ramona, an assertive, demanding first-born child and Gene, a first-born pleaser. Ramona had a violent temper and constantly abused her husband verbally and even physically. It wasn't hard to trace

Ramona's behavior back to how her mother had treated her father.

Ramona had grown up in a family where her mother and dad argued and even exchanged physical blows. It was a very volatile relationship, but her mother usually triumphed. Her mother was extremely strong, ambitious, and materialistic. She was also extremely critical and very unhappy. The father was not ambitious, had few expectations, and lived a detached life. Ramona's mom ran the show.

With that kind of role model, it is not too difficult to understand why Ramona turned out the same way. Instinctively she found herself a man she could dominate and control. In counseling, Gene described himself as "confident on the outside, trembling on the inside." He described his father as a very cold and controlling type who had little time for him.

During a marriage of over twenty-one years, Gene and Ramona had six children. A first born and a pleaser who could never satisfy his father, Gene felt that he was just getting more of the same in his own family. Everything he tried to do met with criticism from Ramona.

After a few counseling sessions, Ramona's problem was clear. She was really angry with her father because he never could stand up to her mother. As I mentioned earlier, in a marriage, one spouse may often turn out to be a scapegoat who has to bear the brunt of his or her mate's anger toward a parent or some other person. This was the case with Gene and Ramona. Gene represented to Ramona everything her father wasn't. Every time he tried to do something, she automatically pulled the rug out from under him. What Ramona really wanted was to have Gene stand up to her. Then she could respect him, something she could never do with her own father because he had continually been bullied by her mother.

One of the major problem areas for Gene and Ramona was sex. Ramona controlled everything in this area and had very specific rules and regulations that Gene had to obey. For example, there would be no foreplay, the light would always have to be out, and there would be no kissing during intercourse. In fact, when Gene was allowed to kiss Ramona, it had to be a tiny peck on the cheek.

Obviously, any sexual relationship that Gene and Ramona managed to have was extremely plastic and detached. There was no spontaneity because everything had to be scheduled. Gene literally had to make an appointment.

Remember that Gene grew up in a family where he was taught not to express his feelings and where his father and his mother were very critical of him. So how did Gene respond to Ramona's tight control in the sexual area? You guessed it. After twenty-one years and fathering six kids, Gene got fed up with Ramona's ridiculous demands. He became impotent. There was nothing wrong with Gene physically, but he articulated his anger and disappointment in the only way he could. He was saying, "Hey, lady, you are totally unfair and I can't get excited about you." Why couldn't Gene simply tell Ramona that? In addition to her anger and volatile temper, Ramona was far more verbal than Gene. She also knew something about psychology and would inundate him with psychological jargon, constantly beating him to the punch verbally. Gene just clammed up. He couldn't handle Ramona.

It all boiled down to a classic struggle (perhaps *classic persecution* would be a better term) between a dominating, abusive woman who believed she only counted when she won and controlled and a first-born pleaser who believed he only counted in life when he could avoid conflict and criticism.

Gene wanted a wife who could be a friend, someone he could have spontaneous fun with, particularly in bed. He ended up with a female buck sergeant who insisted that he approach her like a rat through a maze: "Turn right here, left there, and go straight ahead when I tell you."

This couple was headed for divorce court's door and firm measures were needed. One day I told Gene, "One thing I've learned about powerful people is that they do respect power. You're going to have to do an about-face and make some radical changes if you're going to make any headway with Ramona. You're going to have to stand up to her."

Not long after, Ramona and Gene got into one of their frequent arguments, but this time the outcome was different. They almost came to blows and Gene turned the tables. He told Ramona to get out. He literally pulled her out of the house as he told her he had had it!

I never advise my clients to use violence, but in this case Gene's actions were exactly what their marriage needed. What Ramona had been asking for all the time was that Gene take the lead. She wanted her man to be strong. She used terrible tactics to get him to show strength, but when he finally did, she responded.

From that point, we were able to work with Gene and Ramona on a positive basis. Their problems didn't go away overnight, but they eventually made progress. One key to that progress was helping Ramona realize that when she tried to control and dominate Gene, she was simply reliving her parents' marriage. As soon as Ramona relaxed some of her rigid and ridiculous controls regarding sex, Gene's impotence vanished. The last time I heard, they had even made love with the night-light on!

Not all controllers use Ramona's violence and verbal pyrotechnics. Controllers can also be shy, quiet, sneaky, sweet, syrupy, etc. Controllers are close cousins to perfectionists, but while perfectionists are their own worst enemies, controllers are the enemies of others as well as themselves.

My suggestions to a couple suffering controller problems include the following:

1. *If you are married to a controller, realize you are not going to change your spouse.* You can only change your own behavior and way of interacting and then allow your spouse to decide to change.

2. *Try being positive, but refuse to play your spouse's controlling games.* Pleasantly but firmly refuse to be controlled. If you can force the controller's hand, he or she must act differently, because the payoff is no longer there. The key is to let the controller know that if he wants to control himself, he is welcome. But when he tries to control everyone else in the family, something has to give.

3. *When I have opportunity to counsel a controller, I concentrate on how futile it is to try to control everyone and everything.* It simply doesn't work. In marriage it all comes back to what I said earlier about two being one: When two are one, *both* are in control, *both* are free to do their thing.

Lying Life Lines Shorten Marriages

Today's statistics tell us that the average marriage lasts seven years. No marriage will get very far if one or both spouses have to keep telling themselves lies like the ones we have looked at in this chapter:

"I only count when I'm perfect."
"I only count when I avoid conflict and make peace."
"I only count when I'm noticed and get attention."
"I only count when I am in control."

When counseling married couples, I try to get them to abandon life lines that begin with, "I only count when" and use terminology such as, "I count because." I believe that every husband and wife counts simply because he or she is a human being made in the image of God. If they insist on using, "I only count when" thinking, I suggest, "Tell yourself you can really count when you help your spouse grow and mature as another human being."

What Is Your Favorite Life Line?

There are many more life lines than the ones discussed in this chapter. Listed below are six more variations of or additions to "I only count when I am perfect, avoid conflict, am noticed, or in control." With each life line is a brief analysis and suggestions for how to cope with it.

"I only count when I perform."

This could be a life line for a perfectionist or someone who needs attention. It would depend on what you mean by "perform." Perfectionists have to realize they could never do it all and that their true worth lies in who they are as persons, not in what they do as performers. As for people needing attention, they perform in order to be noticed, applauded, given another carrot. This is selfish behavior and very frustrating because you never get enough carrots!

"I only count when I win."

Obviously this is a variation of, "I only count when I control." Another way to describe this life-style is "win-lose." There's a lot of talk to-day about succeeding and winning, but living by the win-lose code is a constant burden and has-sle. I like to say that winning isn't everything—helping others win is everything.

"I only count when I suffer."

This is the favorite line of people with a mar-tyr complex. They have developed avoiding conflict and making peace at any price into a fine art. Their favorite payoff is to have people say, "Oh, Marian, I don't know *how* you do it."

"I only count when I'm cared for."

This is a hybrid that relates back to, "I only count when I'm noticed," or "when people pay attention." It is a typical life line of a last born, especially a baby princess who is used to being spoiled, cared for, and having her older brothers protect her.

"I only count when I please."

This is a favorite line of the first-born perfectionist who grows up never failing to obey Mommy and Daddy. But in a marriage, a pleaser must always be wary of overdoing it, especially if he or she is married to a controller or a perfectionist. Marriage is a give-and-take proposition. When one person has to do all the giving, it takes its toll on the relationship.

"I only count when I serve God."

I often counsel religious persons who equate sincere belief with "being busy for the Lord." People with a natural tendency to feel they only count when they perform or when they please can quickly burn out in a church because they wind up doing all the work!

Part Five

Birth Order and Parenting: Never Treat Them All the Same

No discussion of birth order would be complete without giving parents some practical help for the daily task of rearing their children. In the final chapters of *The Birth Order Book*, we'll take a look at . . .

- why you should never treat all kids the same
- how Reality Discipline can make your day (and sometimes save it!)
- tips for parenting perfectionists—particularly first borns and only children

- the two-child family and its special pressures
- helping middle children feel less squeezed and more loved
- handling those charming manipulators— the family babies

Chapter Ten

Why Reality Discipline Works With Any Birth Order

How much do you love your children?

Now how is a parent supposed to answer that one? A great deal? Quite a bit? A 9.98 out of a possible 10.00?

Only psychologists ask questions such as, "How much do you love your children?" But let me ask you another one that may be more useful: Do you love your children enough to discipline them?

Notice I said *discipline* and not *punish.* I counsel hundreds of kids and their parents every year. I speak to thousands of parents, teachers, and workers with children at seminars and conventions. I talk about a lot of things, including birth order, but I have only one basic theme:

Love your kids enough to train them with Reality Discipline.

If anything is missing in today's families, it is a system or a strategy for applying consistent, loving discipline to the children. I see the fruits of inconsistency and lack of discipline almost daily in my office.

Parents come to me and ask questions like these:

"What can I do to motivate Richard? He has so much potential, but he just doesn't seem to care."

"We're scared. Lisa is drinking an awful lot and running with the wrong crowd. What can we do?"

"What shall we do with Billy? He just doesn't listen to us anymore. He's downright rebellious and his language is abusive."

"Our Sherry is smoking pot and is brazen about it. She sees nothing wrong. How can we get her to stop?"

My answer always revolves around the same theme. You need to guide your children with the action-oriented techniques of Reality Discipline. And what, exactly, is Reality Discipline? I spent one entire book describing it: *Making Children Mind Without Losing Yours.* In the foreword I described Reality Discipline in general terms:

Action-oriented discipline is based on the reality that there are times—sometimes several per day—when you have to pull the rug out and let the little "buzzards" tumble. I don't mean that literally, of course, but when I talk about pulling the rug out, I mean disciplining a child in such a way that he accepts responsibility and learns accountability for his actions.[1]

What's Your Style of Parenting?

Another way to look at all this is to analyze your parenting style. I see three major approaches being used in families today:

1. authoritarian
2. permissive
3. authoritative

The authoritarian parent is the one who believes he knows what is best for his children. Many parents of my generation grew up in authoritarian homes. If that was your experience, you remember quite clearly that you didn't have a lot of input. You did as you were told and you kept quiet. And if you didn't obey orders and keep quiet, you got the switch.

I can recall chatting with a TV personality when I was "resident psychologist" on her talk-variety show. We were talking about birth order and as a first born, she remembered well the many pressures that were on her to perform and "be perfect." And when she wasn't perfect, she was given the assignment to go out and cut her own switches from the limbs of trees or bushes, bring them back to her father, and submit to a good tanning. Needless to say, this lady grew up in an authoritarian home.

In homes where parents are permissive, we see the child doing just about what he likes:

"Oh, Johnny, honey, would you like to go to bed now or would you rather stay up and watch the eleven o'clock news with us?"

"Oh, that's all right, dear. Let little Jennifer play with the Hummel—she likes it." Permissive parents use an interesting form of logic which says, "If I let little Festus do his own thing, he will love me and always act like a nice little boy."

Of course the opposite is true. Permissive parenting turns out little tyrants who run the house. Permissive parenting *causes* rebellion, rather than preventing it, because the children feel anger and even hatred toward their parents for lack of guidelines and limit setting.

In many homes, however, there is still another problem called "inconsistency." It's quite typical for parents to be permissive—to a point. Then, following their natural instincts, they finally blow their cool. They crack down with a vengeance and authoritarianism reigns supreme for anywhere from a few minutes to a few weeks. And so the children never quite know what to expect.

On the other hand, children learn to play the game. They learn how far to push Mom and Dad. They learn just what decibel Mom's voice can reach before they are in the "red danger zone." As I say in *Making Children Mind* . . . , parental inconsistency is a great way to jerk a kid around (that is, raise a yo-yo).

But there is a third parenting style and I believe it's the answer to our problem. We can stop the inconsistent swing between authoritarianism and permissiveness by standing on the middle ground that I call *authoritative* parenting. It's unfortunate that authoritative sounds so much like *authoritarian,* because people get them mixed up. There is, however, a world of difference in the two approaches. Authoritative parents don't dominate their children and make all decisions for them. And they certainly don't let the children dominate them and make all the decisions for the family. Instead, authoritative parents use the principles of Reality Discipline, which are tailor-made to help them give their children loving correction and training.[2]

How Authoritative Parenting Works

In *Making Children Mind* . . . I illustrate how authoritative parenting works with the example of the seven-year-old who breaks a toy belonging to another child. What should the parent do? One obvious choice would be a good swat, or maybe even a good hard spanking, if this has been a regular pattern of behavior. Another obvious choice might be sending the child to his room, or grounding him for a week. I don't believe any of those choices is the best one. I think the kind of discipline needed in this situation is one based on reality, and reality says if you break someone's else's property, you pay for it.

How can a seven-year-old child pay for a toy? Out of his allowance or piggy bank. Allowances, by the way, are one of the best techniques any parent has for teaching Reality Discipline. It is absolutely amazing how early in life children become financial experts. Even the youngest child soon understands the concept of "the bottom line." When the consequences of his actions start coming out of his own pocket, he immediately starts to really think about what he is doing and why.[3]

How Reality Discipline Can Save Your Day

There is a great deal more to Reality Discipline, and if you want the full story, you will have to get a copy of *Making Children Mind Without Losing Yours*. I give you this blatant commercial without apology, because I believe it is truly a sound and sensible solution to *making children mind*. The book goes into many areas that parents are interested in:

It talks about why reward and punishment

don't really work and why love and encouragement do.

It explains the difference between discipline and punishment.

It gives practical steps any parent can take to teach children how to be accountable and responsible.

It shows you how to "pull the rug out and let the little buzzards tumble"—that is, move in and apply Reality Discipline where it is really needed.

It talks about those times when pulling the rug out might mean using a swat. Yes, I believe in spanking but I think there are usually other more useful and effective means of disciplining before resorting to applying pain to the bum-bum. There are times when a good swat is by far the best discipline at the moment, but the trick is to know when to use the swat and when to use some other approach.

Making Children Mind Without Losing Yours contains countless ideas for dealing with kids—everything from temper tantrums to battles over bedtime, from dealing with lying and fighting to getting them to do their homework and get up in the morning. For our purposes in the remaining chapters of this book, however, I want you to get acquainted with the basic principles and distinctives of Reality Discipline, which include the following:

1. *Reality Discipline is the best system I know to*

avoid inconsistent meandering between authoritarianism and permissiveness. Most parents know instinctively that they should be authoritative—in charge but reasonable and fair. Staying with the authoritative happy medium is best done through Reality Discipline.

2. *Parents never seek to punish; they always seek to discipline, train, and teach.* In the long run, discipline will be more effective than punishment.

3. *Reality Disciplinarians use guidance rather than force, but they are action oriented, not satisfied to use just words.* If "punishment" pain or some kind of consequence is involved, the parent is not doing it or causing it—reality is. Your child is learning how the real world works.

4. *Reality Disciplinarians hold their children accountable for their actions, whatever those actions are, to help their children learn from experience.* That experience may include failure *or success,* but *in all cases the children are responsible and accountable for what they do.*[4]

5. *Above all, Reality Discipline is your best bet for avoiding what I call the Super Parent syndrome.* Super Parents are powerful role models who teach their children that they dare not fail. And of course when parenting the child who has tendencies toward perfectionism (as we will see in the next chapter on parenting the first-born and only child), this can cause real problems.[5]

Never Treat Them All The Same

Oh, yes, one more thing. I firmly believe that parents should never treat all their children exactly the same. Each of your children is different. Each birth order is different. You have to treat each birth order with certain distinctive techniques and understandings. I'm not suggesting you baby anyone or treat one child more fairly than another. In fact, when you use Reality Discipline and treat each child differently according to his needs, it is the only way you can be sure you are being entirely fair!

The key is having a strategy for dealing with each child—each birth order, if you please. In the following chapters we will be looking at how to parent first borns and only children—the ones who are most likely to fall into the trap of perfectionism that I described earlier in this book as "slow suicide."

We'll look at the two-child family—especially that second child and how he branches off from the first. We'll also take a good look at how the second child dethrones the first born and what we can do to make that less traumatic for number one.

We'll also look at the middle child. Middle children are those born anywhere between the first and the last. The big problem for the child born in the middle is that he often feels squeezed, like a fifth wheel who was born too late to get the privileges of the first born and too soon to get the babying and coddling he sees the last born enjoying almost every day.

And the last borns have their challenges, too. Yes, they do get babied and coddled, but they also get treated like "second-class citizens" who are never quite big enough, fast enough, or smart enough to keep up with the others. Last-born children desperately need the encouragement and assurance that they do count and that they can make a contribution.

So, let's get on with our look at how to parent the different birth orders. There are problems and pitfalls to be avoided, but there are also achievements, accomplishments, and joys to be had as we understand the uniqueness of each of our children and how to help them become the complete persons God intended them to be.

How to Be Your Child's Best Friend

Before we start looking at parenting the various birth orders, here are nine tips for making children mind. I like to call them the nine ways you can be your child's best friend.

1. The discipline should fit the infraction. For example, the child misuses his allowance. When he asks for something extra before the week is out, you simply say, "Sorry, you will have to use

your allowance and if you haven't any left, you will have to wait until Saturday."

2. Never beat or bully your child into submission. Remember, the shepherd's rod was used to guide the sheep, not to wale them.

3. Use action-oriented methods whenever possible.

4. Always try to be consistent.

5. Emphasize order and the need for order. Work comes before play, chores come before breakfast, and so on. This concept reinforces obedience and emphasizes that in all of God's kingdom, there is a need for order—order is important.

6. Always require your child to be accountable and responsible for his or her own actions.

7. Always communicate to your child that he or she is good, even though the behavior may have been irresponsible.

8. Always give your child choices that reinforce cooperation but not competition.

9. If spanking is necessary, it should be done when you're in control of your emotions. It should *always* be followed up with explanations for why the spanking was necessary, and those all-powerful words, "I love you and I care about you."[6]

Chapter Eleven

Parenting the Perfectionist: Tips for Rearing First-Born and Only Children

Back in chapters 3, 4, and 5, we talked a good deal about first borns and only children and the major burden they carry through life:

Perfectionism

I know there are moms and dads who will disagree with me on that one. They tell me about first-born Harlan, who is presently seventeen years old and has yet to make his first conscientious move. In fact, he hasn't moved to make his bed in the last six months.

Or a mother will say, "Come on, Dr. Leman. My first-born daughter, Driscilla, is so laid back I have to put a mirror in front of her nose to be sure she's alive. She's getting straight $C-$ in history and math and $A+$ in MTV."

But I still stick by my theory for two very

good reasons: Mom and Dad. Parents of first borns and only children should always ask, "Who were the child's role models during the first months and years of life?" The obvious answer is *they* were. When you are little and try to imitate someone so much older and bigger, you soon get the idea you have to be "perfect."

As they lovingly parented Harlan and Driscilla, Mom and Dad planted seeds of perfectionism without even trying. Now that the children are older they may not look like perfectionists or even act like perfectionists, but the logical explanation is that they are discouraged. Slobs and poor students are often discouraged perfectionists who have given up trying because it hurts too much to fail.

Frank, the Discouraged Twelve-Year-Old

Another question for every parent is, "How perfectionistic am I? What kind of expectations do I have for my child?"

Put an impressionable, conscientious child with exacting, perfectionist parents and you have the makings of a discouraging situation indeed. That was the case with twelve-year-old Frank, son of a father who was a surgeon and a mother who was a registered nurse. With highly

217

educated, exacting parents like those, Frank had to be a perfectionist.

Frank's major problem, supposedly, was a very short temper. He explained to me that he would get up in the morning and carefully plan his day. Most twelve-year-olds can't plan the next fifteen minutes, but Frank knew what he wanted to do from morning until night! He had learned this behavior from his parents, particularly his dad, a surgeon who was a great believer in planning and scheduling everything.

Interestingly enough, Frank was not a true first-born or only child. He was the second of two children, but born seven years after his older brother. As we saw in chapter 2, any time you get that much distance between children, a new "family" can start. With high-powered professionals for parents and seven years between him and his brother, Frank really fit perfectly into the first-born category.

In fact, he could have easily passed for an only child because he had a very difficult time getting along with children his own age. You see, the other kids didn't know or care about Frank's plans for the day. They weren't interested in his "to do" lists. And when Frank's day didn't go right (which was often) he would blow his top. He would pick up his marbles and go home. For example, he played soccer, but if he made one or two errors or mistakes, he'd take himself out of the game. He simply couldn't deal with failure.

The same thing would happen at home. If someone missed an appointment, failed to telephone, or some other "catastrophe" messed up his plan for the day, Frank kicked things, threw things, and even put holes through the walls of the house. On one occasion he severely abused the family dog.

All of this negative behavior really bothered a conscientious boy like Frank. He felt terribly guilty about the way he was acting, but he was trapped in his own carefully planned prison of perfectionism.

I began working with Frank by helping him see that no one can get through the day without a mistake or failure of some kind. Keying on his athletic interests, I pointed out that Babe Ruth hit 714 home runs, but he also struck out 1,330 times!

Frank got the message, and so did his dad. The father, who was Frank's hero, was courageous enough to start admitting his own faults and imperfections, which he had kept carefully hidden over the years. All this helped Frank make tremendous progress with his short temper. While he remained a perfectionist in many ways, Frank saw that he couldn't control everything and that even the best-laid plans were bound to go astray now and then. He wound up being a much happier kid because he stopped trying to do everything the hard way. Most important, Frank learned he didn't have to be perfect to win his father's approval and love.

The Biggest Crisis First Borns Face

"Doing it the hard way" is typical of perfectionists. First borns and only children can easily see life as a struggle—a test or a race they have to win. Later in this chapter we'll look at some specific things you can do to help your first-born or only child in that battle with perfectionism. We'll also share some things that can help you if you are a "perfectionist Super Parent."

First, however, I want to take a substantial look at what I call the biggest crisis any first-born child has to face. And that crisis is very real. I am talking about the reality of "dethronement," which occurs with the arrival of a new little brother or sister.

First borns are the center of attention for a relatively long time, as time is measured in a young child's life. In chapter 9 I mentioned the "style of life" every child develops by age five or so. If Mommy and Daddy don't have a second child until the first born is three years old, realize that three-fifths—*60 percent*—of the first born's style of life has already been formed before the intruder comes home from the hospital. A great part of that style of life has taught the first born that he or she is kingpin. One of the most challenging tasks of parenting is preparing the first-born child for the intrusion of the second.

I always advise parents to let their first-born youngster hold the new baby, feed it, even diaper it, if possible. I know the diaper may look a bit askew, but it's important to get the first born involved. If nothing else, let your first born "go get the box of diapers for Mommy."

Another excellent strategy is to pay particular attention to your first-born child just before the arrival of number two. Do some special things with the first born, such as the following:

1. Have the oldest child put away some of his special toys in a safe place so the baby can't get them. This may sound silly to an adult, but to a three-year-old it makes excellent sense.

2. Reassure the number-one child that Mommy and Daddy will never run out of hugs and kisses after number two arrives. There will be plenty for everyone.

3. Let number-one child choose some toys to give to number two. These toys might be new ones he picks out at the store, or they might be old toys that he is willing to give away.

When the second-born child comes home from the hospital, it will soon draw on the first born that the "thing" is not temporary, that it is going to stay. Now it's doubly important to give the first born some special attention of his own. One good conversational tack is to talk to the first born about all the things the newborn *can't do.*

"[Baby's name] can't even catch a ball, he can't walk, can't talk, can't do anything."

Make a big thing about the newborn having to go to bed while the older child gets to stay up. ("You're three years old—you don't have to go to bed yet. You get to stay up late with Mommy and Daddy.")

Dethronement is never a simple or easy matter. No matter how many precautions parents take, the first born can't help wondering, *Why, wasn't I good enough?* An episode in our own first born's struggle with dethronement is recorded in color on "Super 8" film. The epic scene shows Sande and Kevin proudly posing with newborn Krissy while Grandma runs the camera. None of us—not even my mother—noticed eighteen-month-old Holly as she slipped into the picture, smiling broadly as she dug her elbow into Krissy's midsection.

Later, when we got the film back and rolled the projector, our reaction was ambivalent. Holly's elbow toss was cute and amusing, but it was also a graphic demonstration of how first borns feel dethroned and will make some perfectly natural (selfish) moves to regain their "fair share" of attention from parents.

The first born's natural inclination toward self-ishness is why I want to insert a word of caution about giving your oldest child special treatment to balance things out because there is a new little intruder in the house. Don't ever let the first born manipulate you to get special advantages or to trick you into spoiling him. Reality Discipline always sticks to its guidelines and is consistent. Don't ever give a first born any kind of payoff for a temper tantrum or outbursts of tears. If necessary, isolate the first born for a brief time and then go in and talk about it.

Always follow up discipline with lots of hugging, touching, and talking, and in this case underline and emphasize the first born's advantage over the new baby because he can do so many more things than the baby can. At every opportunity, enumerate the things the first born can do that baby can't. You'll be laying groundwork for a cooperative first-born child. He or she will get through the dethronement crisis more easily because he will know he is more capable, bigger, stronger, and so on.

Being First Doesn't Mean "Be Perfect"

While it's good strategy to shore up the dethroned first-born child's ego by telling him he's bigger, stronger, and knows the ropes better than his little brother or sister, always be aware that you are talking to a perfectionist. Your first born started being a perfectionist long before your second child arrived. Very early—even during his first year—the first born starts to pick up on his adult role models—Mommy and Daddy—and starts setting his sights on being just like them. That includes being just as capable as they are, which is obviously impossible for a tiny child.

This first born's desire to follow in Mommy's and Daddy's footsteps usually increases as the parents give the first born a lot of extra attention—or overparenting. They tend to be overprotective and, of course, they unconsciously push the child to accomplish everything he can (and some things he can't). It's no wonder first borns walk and talk earlier than any other birth order, they have a larger vocabulary, etc. First borns, along with their perfectionist cousins the only children, grow up being "little adults." Part of their adult behavior is that they become very obedient to authority, another holdover from trying to please the two key authority figures in life—mother and father.

A first born may set great store by authority and power because of a dethronement experience he may have suffered. Dr. Alfred Adler, who was a pioneer in birth order studies, claimed that when a child loses his power and the small kingdom that was his for the several years before second-born brother or sister arrived, he understands better than other people the importance of power and authority and how precious it really is. As grown-ups, first borns may exaggerate the importance of rules and laws. They believe everything should be done by the book and the book should never be changed or rewritten.

You can find a classic example of this in the New Testament parable of the prodigal son. The younger son (apparently the baby in the family) took his share of the inheritance early and went out to live it up. The elder son, however, stayed with his father and obediently tended the flocks and the fields. When the younger boy finally came to his senses and returned home, the father was so pleased and thankful that he threw a big bash, complete with the fatted calf. The elder son came up from the field (where else would an elder son be but working in the fields?) and when he heard all the revelry he became incensed. He just couldn't understand how his younger brother could go blow it all and then come home to a big banquet, with lots of gifts, like rings and robes. And here he had stuck it out on the old homestead with shoulder to wheel and nose to grindstone. And what had he gotten for his trouble? Not once had his father ever thrown a banquet for him—not even a little party.[1]

Typically, parents enforce stricter rules and regulations with their first born than they will with later-born children. You see, they want to do it right with this first child, so they keep a tight rein on him. This is why I feel it is vital that parents develop an *authoritative* style of parenting combined with the techniques of Reality Discipline. The authoritative parent is loving and fair but also consistent and firm. The authoritative parent is the happy medium between the two extremes that can do a child so much harm: authoritarianism and permissiveness.

Nicole: Lying Was the Easy Way Out

People often ask me which style of parenting is more harmful: the authoritarian or the permissive. I really can't give the nod to one or the other. I see both problems almost weekly in my office.

Nicole was fourteen when her parents brought her to me for counseling due to what they called "rebellion." She had been suspended from school for cutting classes and smoking pot. As I talked with Nicole she told me her parents allowed her very little freedom and they made almost every choice for her. They not only picked out her clothes but they told her how to wear them, when she could go out, when she could come in. They literally controlled how she spent every minute of her days.

Of course, the more the parents pushed, the more Nicole withdrew and rebelled. In such an authoritarian environment, it was easy for Nicole to learn to lie. The child learns to tell the parents what they want to hear. When this happens, the child develops two lives. There was the Nicole who lived around her mother and father and there was another kind of Nicole who ran with her peer group.

Because Nicole had been so controlled all her life, she really didn't know how to think for herself when it came to being pressured by her peer group. Nicole's friends got the best of her and she became involved in using drugs and alcohol, along with behaving promiscuously with the boys in her school. As I counseled Nicole, I learned that her "game plan" was to turn eighteen, get out of the house, buy a car, and split.

Nicole was a first-born child with a younger sister, who was eleven, and a younger brother, who was eight. Nicole was also a defeated perfectionist. Her mother was an ultraperfectionist who kept the home impeccably neat. Nothing was ever out of place. Even Nicole kept her room immaculate at all times, a rather odd behavior for someone as rebellious as she. However, it fit in with her "I'll tell them what they want to hear" behavior, which was the front she used at home to hide her wild life with the peer group.

Nicole's mother was the key to the perfectionism in that home. She "wore the pants" in the family, and told everyone what to do, including the father, who was a long-distance truck driver.

It was not too difficult to see why Nicole rebelled the way she did (and why Dad was a long-distance truck driver). I worked with Nicole and her parents for six weeks. Progress was slow at first because her mother and father didn't want to listen and they had to be encouraged to let Nicole talk. Nicole was afraid to admit the truth about running with a wild crowd, drinking, using drugs, and engaging in sex. She was sure her parents would shut her down completely, or not even want to have her in their home anymore.

Fortunately, Nicole's parents were not beyond hope as far as their authoritarian ways were concerned. They did listen and they learned. We finally made some progress and at the end of six weeks I had Nicole write a summary of the positive things that had come out of her counseling. Here's what she said:

> I think my mom and dad are willing to give me some freedom now. I think they understand that I am me and not them. I don't think we will fight as much. I really want to know my parents, I want them to

get to know me. I know it is not going to be easy for them to trust me anymore, but I am willing to be patient and wait until that day comes as well. I know I have caused a lot of grief and problems and I know that part of this problem comes from my having to lie. I always felt like I had to lie because if I told the truth I would get into trouble and they would never let me do anything. So I have made the commitment to listen. Together we have been able to pull things off so far. Mom and Dad are giving me more leeway and I am not lying to them. I am being honest with them and it makes me feel good being honest.

Nicole was a classic example of a first-born child who had grown up watching her mom and dad and who actually wanted to imitate them, up to a certain age. But the authoritarian treatment her parents gave her as she moved into the teenage years was too much. She became a defeated perfectionist, and turned to wild and crazy behavior as a way of crying for help.

Nicole is a good example of why no parent should ever think a first-born child is not a perfectionist simply because that first-born child isn't toeing the mark, keeping his room clean, or obeying all the rules. The child may be breaking all the rules because he or she is, in fact, a perfectionist who can't handle the cards life is dealing at the moment.

Perfectionists Don't Need "Model" Parents

The way we psychologists sometimes go on with our advice, it sounds as if we are trying to turn our listeners and readers into model parents who never make mistakes. If I have said anything that sounds like that, forgive me. Actually I believe that no child in any birth order needs "model parents" or what I also call "Super Parents." First borns and only children in particular have enough problems trying to be perfect and fail-safe without coping with parents who literally never make mistakes. Actually, there are few, if any, parents who never *make* mistakes, but there are a lot of them who refuse to *admit* it!

Has your three-year-old first born or only child ever heard you say, "I blew it. I was wrong. I forgot. I'm sorry"? Has your *thirteen-year-old* ever heard you say any of those things freely and openly? A lot of parents choke on those words, especially if they are first-born or only-child perfectionists themselves.

If you are something of a perfectionist, remember that your child needs encouragement more than prodding. Learn to simply hold your child when he or she is having problems. Just say, "Everything's going to be okay. What's the problem? You say this isn't working out right. Would you like me to help?"

Remember Marilou, the little perfectionist who had fits of temper because she messed up cutting out perfect circles as a preschooler and who went on to having fits of temper when her husband forgot to hold up his end of the housework? Marilou could have benefited a great deal from a mom or dad who held the paper as she cut out the circle and said things like, "It's hard, isn't it? I don't always cut perfect ones myself. I remember how hard it was when I was small."

Or take the instance when Mom gets tired of the four-year-old's messy toy box and sends him to his room to clean it up. The problem is that the entire task may look too big to the four-year-old. There are just too many toys and books and crayons and puzzles scattered from one end of the room to the other. How can he possibly get all this done?

What a parent can do in this case is come in and sit down and say, "Honey, there is a lot to do here, so while you pick up your toys I'm going to sit right here and talk to you about what we're going to do tonight."

Chances are, the kid will get on with the job and complete it in fairly good fashion. If he doesn't get everything just right, don't berate him or do it all over for him. *Be satisfied with a less-than-perfect job.* The great temptation for a perfectionist parent is to send messages to the child that say, "Get in there and measure up, kid. You've got to do an absolutely flawless job or I won't approve."

Please be assured I am *not* saying you should let a child get away with goofing off—not doing the job at all. Hold him accountable for his responsibilities; just don't demand that he has to be perfect. Instead, relax your perfectionist rules a bit. If the child has made his own bed and it's wrinkled in spots, congratulate him but don't do it over for him. You can shut the door and no one will see the two or three wrinkles.

Learn to be flexible. Instead of giving orders, help your child do things. Remember, you are the role model for your first born or only child. He has no brother or sister to look to and pattern after. *You* are what he has to pattern after and you are an awesome act to follow! So whenever you can, show him that you are human, that you understand, that you are not perfect, and that mistakes are not the end of the world. In this way you will do a great deal to help your first born or only child become less of a perfectionist who grows up to whip and drive himself with expectations that are far beyond human capacity.

Another way to demonstrate to your first born or only child that you are not invincible is to ask your child for help now and then. I'm not talking about helping with the baby, going to get the diapers for Mommy, and so on. I'm talking about asking your child (and you can do this with even a very young child at the preschool level), "Will you help me decide what to have for dinner tonight?"

Granted, left entirely to his own devices, the youngster might come up with an interesting diet of peanut butter sandwiches, Oreo cookies, and lots of ice cream. But you can head this off by asking if he would prefer chicken or hamburgers. Give him several choices for dessert, and let him choose the one that you will use. (If you don't like Oreo cookies for dessert, don't have them in the house!)

Reality Discipline With First Borns and Onlies

Remember back in chapter 10 when I gave you nine tips for being your child's best friend? Those nine tips all share principles about how to use Reality Discipline with your child. I advise new parents of a first-born child to review them often. The reality of the situation is that parents of a first born are new at all this. I try to encourage them to go easy on turning out the world's first "perfectly behaved child." I can safely say it isn't going to happen anyway. All children misbehave—even mine. To put it an-

233

other way, all children make mistakes—just as their parents do.

If anything, parents should go a little easier on the first-child. I'm not saying that they should be permissive; on the contrary, Reality Discipline is consistent and fair and firm with every child, no matter what the birth order. But what I'm concerned about is this natural parental desire to make the first-born child some kind of guinea pig.

Let's face it, we are learning the ropes with the first born and the tendency is to err on the side of being too strict. Keep that in mind as you discipline your first-born child, no matter what age he or she is right now. And also keep in mind that whatever rules, regulations, and requirements you have set for the first born, be sure those rules and regulations stay the same for the other children as they come along. If you tend to forget what the rules were, just ask your first-born child. He or she will refresh your memory in a hurry!

When disciplining any age level, there is no more important rule than to be fair and consistent. As I have emphasized, parents tend to overparent, overdiscipline, and overpunish the first child. The first born and only child become very, very susceptible to authority, rules, and regulations. Our own daughter, Holly, has a favorite TV program. I'll name three shows and you tell me which one it is:

1. "Little House on the Prairie"
2. "People's Court"
3. "The Waltons"

The correct answer is "People's Court." For Holly, our meticulous perfectionistic first born, the favorite TV hero isn't Magnum or John Boy. She loves to watch Judge Wapner as he arbitrates heavy questions like, "Should the teenager get his money back for the used car because the salesman lied to him?" Holly loves rules, regulations, and legalities. She often gives the same decision that Judge Wapner hands down. I once found a charge of fifty cents on our phone bill and started asking, "Who made this call?" It turned out Holly had placed the call, to give her vote in favor of the plaintiff on "People's Court"!

One good way to be fair with your first born is to not always assume that your oldest child is your built-in baby-sitter. For example, if your first-born daughter (this happens more with girls than boys) is around ten or eleven and you have younger children, ages seven and four, there is a natural convenience in asking little Mildred to watch her brother and sister for a few minutes while you run to the market.

As time goes on, little Mildred is being asked to baby-sit for the evening while you and hubby go to the movies. I'm not saying there aren't times when Mildred couldn't watch the younger kids, but I am saying that it shouldn't become a regular and expected thing. If you want your first born to feel you are being fair, make a special point of allowing him or her to have the evening off now and then. If you need to have the younger children watched, hire a sitter. At least talk with your first-born child about what her plans might be before you assume that she can drop everything and "baby-sit for a few hours."

Of course, it goes without saying that in a family of two or more children the parents should bend over backwards to be as consistent in discipline with the younger children as they were with the first born. The classic stereotype in the typical family of three sees the parents ruling with an iron hand (or at least a wooden switch) with the first child. Then they relax a bit with the coming of the second and by the time the last born shows up they have turned to putty.

Ask almost any first-born child in America and he or she will tell you the baby of the family "gets away with murder." If anything, the last-born child should be disciplined *more* than the first-born and middle children. This is a sensitive issue, however, and we'll look at it more closely in the chapter on parenting the last-born child.

Tips for Parenting First Borns

Besides going over the general principles of Reality Discipline back in chapter 10, here are some particular tips for parenting the perfectionistic first born. These same suggestions apply to only children as well.

1. Don't reinforce your first born's already ingrained perfectionistic tendencies. Don't be an "improver" on everything he says and does. Go easy on reminding the child of what he "should" be like.

2. Realize first borns have a particular need to know exactly what the rules are. Be patient and take time to lay things out for your first born from "A to Z."

3. Recognize the first born's first place in the family. As the oldest, the first born should get some special privileges to go along with the additional responsibilities that always seem to come his way.

4. Take "two on one" time—both parents out with the oldest child alone. First borns respond better to adult company than any other birth order.

5. Stay away from making your first born your "instant baby-sitter." At least try to check with your first born to see if his or her schedule would allow for some baby-sitting later in the day or that evening.

6. As your first born grows older, be sure you don't pile on more responsibilities. Alleviate some responsibilities and give them to the younger children as they are capable of taking these jobs on. One first born told me at a seminar, "I'm the garbage person." By that he meant that he had to do everything at home while his brother and sister got off much easier.

7. When your first born is reading to you and has trouble with a word, don't be so quick to jump in with a correction. First borns are extremely sensitive to criticism and being corrected. Give the child time to sound out the word. Give help when *he* asks for it.

Chapter Twelve

Parenting the Two-Child Family: Two May Be Company . . . or a Crowd

If parenting first borns means preventing discouraged perfectionists, parenting second borns means watching out for rivalries.

Because more and more families are opting for only two children these days, it's well worth our time to take a brief look at the two-child family, with some special attention focused on the second born.

I've always been curious about the birth order of the creator of the well-known Avis Rent-a-Car advertising campaign that ran for years in competition with Hertz, recognized leader in the field. It's my guess he (or she) is a second-born child who understands perfectly that when you're number two you have to try harder!

Rivalry and Role Reversal

In the two-child family especially, there is bound to be rivalry, particularly when the children are the same sex. Whenever a second-born child joins the family, some key principles are always at work. One of these key principles could be stated like this:

> Second-born children develop their own life-style according to the perceptions they have about themselves and the key persons in their lives.

Obviously, a very important person in the second-born child's life is the older sibling. In fact, another rule of thumb is that each child in the family is always most deeply influenced and affected by the one just ahead of him: the only child or first born by the parents; the second child by the first born; the third child by the second born, and so on (see chapter 6).

In chapter 11 we looked at dethronement— the trauma every first born goes through when number two arrives. Sometimes dethronement can be devastating to a first born, in other cases it is more of an inconvenience or irritation. However dethronement affects the first born, it means he or she is no longer the one and only highlight in the life of Mom and Dad. Dethronement is unavoidable, and coming right along with it is an automatic state of rivalry.

There's a natural tendency on the part of the second-born child to look above and see who has been there first. Instinctively, while still very young, the second-born child will decide whether he is going to "go for it" and compete with the first-born child, or whether he will branch off in an entirely different direction and leave certain areas as the first born's exclusive territory. If the second-born child does move in and "take over" with regard to leadership or achievement, we call that a "role reversal." For all practical purposes the second-born child becomes the first born, as far as family roles are concerned.

Some Examples of Role Reversal

Second borns may compete with an older brother or sister in various ways. Some do it quite openly, others are a bit more clever—even sneaky—in trying to reach their goal. Let's take a look at one example where the second born openly took over from the first born and definitely was a better-adjusted person.

I once worked with a two-child family comprised of two girls, close in age. The younger competed openly with her older sister, which really wasn't that difficult. The older girl got kicked out of high school for cutting classes. She drifted from job to job, even had some brushes with the law over drugs. While the first-born girl was fouling things up, the younger sister was putting it all together. With her parents cosigning for her, she had her own charge and checking accounts by age sixteen. She went on to college and got into a promising program working toward a marketing degree. To make matters still worse for the older girl, she got pregnant and had the baby out of wedlock. She lives at home with her parents, who are as distressed by their oldest as they are proud of their youngest.

What we have in this example is a classic case of role reversal. It is also an unhappy illustration of dethronement of the first child by the second. Every first born gets dethroned to some degree with the birth of number two, because number one is no longer "total king or queen of the castle." But first borns can be dethroned more severely if they do not live up to the challenge of being pacesetter in the family.

In our example, the younger girl looked up at her older sister and saw that she was setting a slow pace, going in directions that weren't paying off—always in a hassle with her parents, in trouble at school, etc. The younger sister branched off in the other direction—became a pleaser, good student, and ambitious worker. She wasn't two-faced or manipulative about it; she just openly set out to do her best in holding to the values her parents appreciated. For example, she became known for coming home from college at the end of the school term and saying, "Hey, Mom and Dad, I'm going out to find a summer job. I won't be home until I get one." And she would always have her job before sundown.

Another well-known role reversal is the story of Jacob and Esau in the Old Testament. But in the biblical account we find Jacob, born the second of twins, being sneaky and deceptive, not exactly marks of good adjustment to life.

I sometimes wonder if Isaac and Rebekah didn't make some kind of self-fulfilling prophecy when they named their twin boys. Their first born they called Esau and their second they named Jacob, which means "supplanter" (that is, to usurp the position of another).

Esau, the powerful older brother, was a hairy macho type who spent a lot of time outdoors. Jacob was smoother—in a lot of ways. He hung around the house and was something of a "gentleman of the manor" as well as a gourmet of sorts. He was also his mother's favorite. When Esau came home famished from one of his hunting trips, Jacob saw his chance. Esau asked for some stew that Jacob had just prepared. With the savory smells filling the room, Jacob decided to put a rather high price on Esau's snack time: "How about the birthright in exchange for the stew?" he suggested.

243

For a first born, Esau wasn't exactly strong on critical reflection or thinking things through. He said, "Why not? What good is a birthright if I starve to death?"

Of course, Esau wasn't really starving. He was simply "starved" in the way any of us are starved after heavy exercise outdoors. Jacob got the birthright in trade for a bowl of stew and then tricked his father into giving him the patriarchal blessing as well.[1]

Parenting Two Boys Can Get Lively

In two-child families we generally wind up with a first born and a baby—the conscientious, careful achiever and the charming manipulator. The first born/baby combination holds particularly true if the children are the same sex. If you have a boy and a girl, you have a greater possibility of developing two first borns. The reason for this is that most families have distinctive expectations of how children develop male and female roles. Let's look at a family with two brothers and examine some of the livelier aspects of parenting them.

Rivalry is most intense when you have a two-child family with two boys. Something else to consider, however, is that while two brothers have no trouble learning how to interact with peers of their own sex, they tend to have little preparation for interaction with the opposite sex. The relationship between Mom and her two sons is critical. She is the one who has to do all of the teaching and modeling as to what women are really all about.

It's critical for the mother of two boys to use Reality Discipline—firmly and consistently. She should never—and I mean *never*—take any garbage from them. She should never get into power struggles, or put herself in a position where the boys can walk on her or be disrespectful to her. Why? Because she not only is representing parenthood and motherhood but she's also representing all of womanhood to her two sons. If her two sons learn to walk on her, they'll learn to walk on their wives later. The recent increase in battered wives is really no surprise, and a lot of it can be traced to how the husband learned to relate to women when he was young.

But let's look at the two brothers and examine especially the older brother. Typically, our older brother is going to identify very much with the establishment (Mom and Dad). He is going to be the standard-bearer, the one who picks up on family values and practices them faithfully. He will probably be the leader, and also the family "sheriff" or "policeman" as far as keeping the younger brother in line. Older brother often finds himself being the protector of baby brother.

Older brother usually gets a kick out of having younger brother follow him, and in this very basic way the older boy learns a lot of practical leadership skills. This is a very basic reason you find more first borns in leadership positions in adult life.

At the other end of the family, the younger brother is eyeing older brother and deciding which way he will go. Another key principle that seems to apply in most cases is this:

The second-born child will be the opposite of the first-born, particularly if they are less than five years apart and of the same sex.

The younger child looks the situation over and usually branches off in a different direction. That different direction may still put him in direct rivalry with his older brother. If he is determined to catch up with him and surpass him as far as leadership and achievement are concerned, this can get sticky. For the first-born boy it can get downright devastating, if a true role reversal happens.

Rivalries are most likely to be heated if the boys are closer in age. If there is a three- or four-year spread, the rivalry usually will be less intense and there will be some good leadership on the part of the first-born male. Put them eleven months apart, however, and Mom and Dad may really have their hands full.

When two brothers are born close together,

there is less chance for the older brother to establish a clear superiority. This can be particularly true when physical size comes into play. Younger brother can pull a complete role reversal on older brother due to a sheer height-and-weight advantage.

One of the most graphic examples of role reversal I ever worked with was fifteen-year-old Jimmy and his younger brother, Mike, who at age fourteen was six and one-half inches taller and forty-five pounds heavier than his "big" brother. Throughout their lives Mike had always been bigger, stronger, even faster. All this left Jimmy feeling life had dealt him a very low blow. And it didn't help any when Jimmy's parents cracked down on him much harder than Mike with all kinds of authoritarian rules. At fifteen he had a bedtime of nine o'clock. He got no allowance because he "wasn't responsible." His parents claimed they couldn't trust him and gave him no freedom. Jimmy retaliated by becoming a liar, thief, and possessor of a volatile temper.

When Jimmy was sent to see me he had been putting holes in the wall, smashing windows, and "borrowing" the family car, even though he wasn't old enough to drive. When I got the whole story, my first suggestion to the parents was to loosen the tight reins on Jimmy. Bedtime was made more reasonable for a fifteen-year-old, and he was given an allowance. I also got the

["\n\n\n"]

parents to modify their ironclad rule on "no driving until you're eighteen." Telling the average youngster about to turn sixteen that he can't drive for two more years is sort of like pulling the pin in a grenade and hoping it won't go off. No wonder Jimmy had been "borrowing the car" without permission!

I also helped Jimmy make some progress in dealing with the role-reversal problem by suggesting he stop making so many comparisons between himself and his much larger brother. One thing that also helped was that Mike was a congenial kid who generally liked his older brother and wanted to be like him in some respects. He didn't try to reverse their roles; it simply happened.

Jimmy tried to take my advice on not making so many comparisons, and while he didn't completely rid himself of the sting of the role reversal, he made good progress. His bursts of temper subsided. The lying and cheating stopped and his grades rose from *C*s and *D*s to *A*s and *B*s. The parents were so pleased that not long after he turned sixteen he got his driver's license and particularly enjoyed giving rides to Mike, who was still too young to drive.

Parenting Two Girls Is No Cakewalk

What happens when both children in the two-child family are girls? The basic "same sex" rivalry is there but it probably isn't as intense. Role reversals can occur, however, as demonstrated by the case of the older teenage sister who was completely blowing it as far as the rest of the family was concerned.

In a two-girl family, I believe the father is a key figure. Realize, Dad, the girls are vying for your individual attention. Try to give each daughter as much one-on-one time as you can. In recent years, a lot has been made out of "family time"—those times when everyone goes out together for ice cream or sees a movie. In some cases, family time can mean a special evening at home where the whole family plays games together. While family times are a great idea, they will never replace those times when a child can have Mom or Dad to herself.

While working on this chapter through the evening, I have received the following invitations from my first-born and second-born daughters:

From Holly: "Please come to my room to talk."

From Krissy: "Can I sleep on the floor in your bedroom tonight?"

If I'm wise, I will respond to both notes by

spending some individual time with each child. Little girls often vie for their daddy's attention.

Parents sometimes wonder if granting their children lots of "one-on-one time" actually caters to their selfishness. I say absolutely not. In most families, one-on-one time just isn't that plentiful and when you do spend it, you don't cater to selfishness as much as you build the child's self-esteem and sense of individual worth.

A Boy for You, a Girl for Me

Rivalry between a boy and a girl is usually much less intense, if it exists at all. Let's look, for example, at the older brother/younger sister combination that is three years apart. Three-year-old Horace had to go through a mild dethronement crisis when little Hortense came home from the hospital, but he soon realized Hortense was a girl and not a serious threat to taking over his "turf."

Little guys like Horace seem to have a natural instinct about this. They are also very aware that they get different toys, different clothes, and so on. In most cases, the competition between a boy and a younger sister is not that strong. In fact, a first-born boy and second-born girl can often develop a close emotional bond.

In this kind of combination, little sister usually

grows up to be super feminine. She has Mommy and Daddy and also her big brother all waiting on her, interceding for her, caring for her. This can make for a fairly peaceful family while the two children are growing up, but it can cause trouble for younger sister later, if she becomes too helpless and dependent on men. When this kind of woman gets married, she often winds up disillusioned and an excellent candidate for the classic seven-year marriage.

When the sister is the oldest child, the typical picture is that the little boy has a second mother. This can work out fine, unless the little guy feels that two "mothers" are too much.

I recall working with a boy of fifteen who ran away from home because his mother and older sister "ganged up on me to nitpick." In this case Mom was the chief culprit, but older sister didn't help when she told Johnny, "You're *so* immature!"

Johnny finally came home, after spending a week or so at a friend's house across town. When the family came to me for counseling I learned that Johnny resented how his mom "wore the pants in the family" and dominated him, as well as his quiet, passive father. Fortunately, the mother was wise enough to be willing to learn. After several counseling sessions, in which I encouraged the father to do the talking and leading for a change, we got it worked out. Johnny didn't pull any more runaway capers and eventually wound up helping teach younger kids in his church.

Granted, Johnny's story is something of an extreme case. A more typical scenario finds the older sister and younger brother going their own directions in a much less radical way. If given equal treatment and opportunity, they both take on first-born traits as first-born girl and first-born boy.

That was what happened with my older sister, Sally, and my second-born brother, Jack. Sally was a classic first born: conscientious, well mannered, captain of the cheerleaders in high school, and very popular. She was also an $A+$ student who would drive everyone a little crazy by coming out of tests holding her head and wailing, "I blew it, I know I blew it!"

Two days later, her A was posted at the top of the board.

Jack wasn't quite in Sally's $A+$ league, but he held his own nicely with a $B+$ average in high school, making the Dean's List in college and going on for a Ph.D. He also became an excellent football quarterback in high school and played on his college team as well. Jack always had lots of friends—especially among the young women!

Jack never really competed with Sally that much, and she treated him with a lot of respect—even leading cheers for his football exploits. When they were small, Sally tried "mothering" her little brother (three years younger) on occasion but he never bought into it much. She had a lot better luck when bear cub Kevin came along five years later. I'll talk more about that in chapter 14.

"I'm Not Like My Older Sister"

Whatever combination you come up with, the two-child family is an excellent laboratory for practicing a basic parenting principle: *Accept their differences.*

Of course, we should accept differences no matter how many children are in the family, but there is something about having "only two" that focuses the challenge more sharply. We soon see that we can accept some things more easily than others. For example, when one child is six inches taller than the other, we can accept that. But suppose one child doesn't behave the same or has a completely different set of attitudes and emotions. One child is easy to handle or what a lot of parents like to call "good." The other child is a handful and naturally his behavior gets labeled "bad."

The challenge for parents in cases like this is to realize that each child is different. They must love each child but relate to each child differently. They must maintain some kind of order and consistency in the family and yet always be aware of the individual differences.

Just this week, a nineteen-year-old young lady told me in a counseling session, "I wish you'd tell my mother I'm not like my older sister."

What I heard this girl saying was that her mother was telling her she had to measure up to the standard-bearer in the family: big sister. And because she wasn't making it, she didn't feel accepted in life. If there is anything we can and must do as parents it's to give each of our children unqualified love that is not determined by how good their grades are, how well they perform at home, or anything else. The challenge is to just love each child for who he or she is.

If you can pull that off, the two-child family can really be a breeze. Think of all the advantages: The whole family fits better in the average car. When you all go out to a restaurant you don't have to wait as long. Most restaurant booths are made for four.

Tips for Parenting the Two-Child Family

As with all birth orders, you should first review the principles of Reality Discipline in chapter 10. What is particularly important with a two-child family is to put emphasis on consistency and fairness. For example:

1. Are bedtimes different for the children? Even if the difference is as little as half an hour, it's important that that difference be enforced. Your first born is watching. . . .

2. Are responsibilities and allowances also different? The rule is this: Oldest child gets the most allowance and the most responsibility, but as we said earlier, don't pour it on the oldest child. Be sure the younger one holds up his end.

3. Avoid comparisons. That is easy for a psychologist to advise, hard to do in day-to-day living. Be aware of the dangers of those famous words, "Why aren't you like your brother [or sister]?" Obviously, one child is *not* like his brother or sister and your remark is not only damaging, it is a foolish waste of breath.

4. Don't feel compelled to do for one what you did for the other. In other words, treating each child differently may mean that sometimes one child "gets a little more" than the other. It all evens out in the end.

5. Do things with one child at a time. In other words, give both children plenty of one-on-one opportunities. How can you find time in your busy schedule to do this? You don't *find* it: you *make* it. Take one child alone on a shopping trip, or even a business trip. If possible, leave half an hour early in the morning and stop for a quiet breakfast before dropping him or her off at

school. Dozens of ways to spend one-on-one time will occur to you, if you really *want to do it.* Just remember the cardinal rule: Whatever you do with one child, do with the other.

Chapter Thirteen

Parenting the Middle Child: Taking the Squeeze Off

The middle child at our house is Krissy, currently age thirteen. Not surprisingly, she has been very friendly and outgoing almost since the day she discovered her older sister, Holly, and the reality that she would never have Mom and Dad all to herself.

Krissy's first day at kindergarten was a day my wife will never forget. With some trepidation, Sande put Krissy on the bus, said a "Thank You for taking care of her" prayer, and went back home to try to keep her mind on the morning's tasks.

Meanwhile, Krissy rode down to kindergarten and apparently had a great day. At 11:45 A.M. the kindergarten bus stopped in front of the house and two other little tykes who lived in the neighborhood got off. Krissy did not.

To her credit, Sande waited almost forty-five minutes before she hit the panic button. Surely, she thought, another bus would be along soon.

When none appeared, she called the school. The school informed her that Krissy had gotten on the bus and they couldn't understand why she didn't get off at her own house.

At this point, Sande forgot all about keeping up appearances and looking as if she had child rearing under control. She went a little crazy. She started calling everyone she could think of to ask if they had seen Krissy. Between calls, the phone rang:

"Hi, Mom, this is Krissy."

"Krissy! Where *are* you?"

"I'm at my best friend's house."

"Honey, *where are you? Whose* house are you at?"

Krissy put down the phone. "What's your name again?" Sande could hear her saying.

It turned out that "what's her name" was Jennifer—a little girl Krissy had met for the very first time that very first day in kindergarten. Jennifer's house was on the way home and Krissy had decided to get off the bus and visit awhile with her new friend. It had never occurred to her that Mom might be worried when she didn't get off the bus at our stop. She wasn't trying to be disrespectful, she was simply being her easygoing, sociable self.

Actually, Krissy started her laid-back, going along with life even earlier than kindergarten. I can recall an eighteen-month-old Krissy "swimming" with the aid of "floaties" attached to her shoulders. Older kids were all over the pool, diving, splashing, making waves, and Krissy was out in the middle of it, just enjoying life.

It seems Krissy has always gone along with everything, a very easygoing, friendly sort who could become "best friends" in one morning at kindergarten. Holly, her older sister, has taken the much more serious approach to things that is typical of perfectionists. Holly would *never* get off the kindergarten bus before her stop. She would come straight home no matter what, because *rules are rules.* Holly lives by the code that all conscientious people know instinctively. She is quiet, thoughtful, an excellent student, and a voracious reader. Krissy is like her father. It's an effort to read anything. There's too much of life out there waiting to be tasted and enjoyed. Krissy would rather read people than books. Holly has friends, but her closest friends are books.

Is Krissy a "typical" middle child? Yes—and no. If you'll recall the list of characteristics for describing middle children (chapter 6) it is riddled with contradictions. For example, middle children are sociable, friendly, and outgoing. Krissy certainly fits all three. But, a lot of middle children are also characterized as loners, quiet and shy. Many middle children take life in stride with a laid-back attitude. That's Krissy, most of the time. But under that blithe countenance is a very sensitive little girl who can be as stubborn as an Arizona pack mule when she's riled.

As we noted back in chapter 6, it's harder to get a handle on the middle children than on anyone else in the family. The only child, the firstborn child, and the baby all stick out rather prominently. But the middle child sort of blends in like a quail against the desert floor.

The same principles that apply to the second born are usually equally applicable to the middle child. Like second borns, middle children follow their own version of Murphy's Law:

> I'm going to live according to what I see just above me in the family. I'll size up the situation and then take the route that looks the best.

"Everyone Is Running My Life!"

If any generalizations can be made about middle children it is that they feel squeezed and/or dominated. It's important for parents to be extra aware that the middle child often feels as if "everyone is running my life." Not only does the middle child have a set of parents in authority over him but he has an older sibling right there also. If the older sibling is close in age (within two or three years), the older sibling is almost sure to get in his licks on telling the middle child what to do. And, of course, just below the middle child is the baby of the family, who seems to be getting away with murder. The middle child feels trapped. He is too young for the privileges received by his older brother or sister and he's too old to get away with the shenanigans that are often pulled by the baby in the family.

With these pressures from above and below, middle children wind up feeling like fifth wheels, misfits who have no say and no control. Everyone else seems to be making their decisions while they are asked to sit, watch, and obey.

Sande and I got a taste of how sensitive the middle child can be about parental decisions when Krissy confronted her mother about a class in creative dramatics that Sande had enrolled her in a few days before. Krissy is very much the sensitive type and her little lip jutted out and tears trickled as she let her mother know how unfair it was to sign her up for creative dramatics. I happened to walk in on the conversation so I asked, "But Krissy, do you enjoy dramatics?"

"I love it!" (Sob.)

I laughed and said, "Then why are you getting on Mom's case?"

"You might think it's funny, but I don't think it's so funny. How would you like me to sign Mommy up for swimming lessons?"

I had to think a bit about that one. We have a

backyard pool and Sande gets in it about twice a year to get wet. But I got Krissy's point. She wanted to do her own enrolling in creative dramatics. She didn't need Mommy's help!

So the moral of the story is to take special care to ask your middle child, especially, for his or her opinion, particularly when the decision directly involves him or her. It's important, of course, to ask the opinions of all your children whenever you can because this helps develop their self-esteem and their sense of responsibility and accountability.

Is There Any Hope for the Middle Child?

So far, much of this chapter sounds like a sympathy letter to middle children. Is there any hope for poor little middle-born Milford, who wanders off to find friends because he's a fifth wheel at home? What can parents do with these kids who are such sensitive bundles of contradictions, who supposedly feel squeezed and dominated as adults ignore their opinions and make all their decisions for them?

We have already touched on taking care to allow middle children to take part in decisions that affect them and the family. Another good practice is to go out of the way to make sure middle children feel special. Keep in mind that it can be frustrating to be a middle child. You get a "new" shirt or sweater and find out it's really four years old. Life isn't always that great when you are second or third in line.

One of the ways I make Krissy feel very special is to always make a date to take her to breakfast on her birthday. If you look at my schedule book, you will see that May 16 is always completely cleared of appointments. The reason I clear the day is that it's Krissy's birthday and we start out by going to breakfast together. If it's a school day, I take her to breakfast and later I pick her up for lunch and take her to one of the classy places in town, like McDonald's.

We really make a big deal out of birthdays at our house. I do the same thing with each child, but I am especially aware of how important it is to Krissy. In fact, the last time Krissy and I had breakfast on her birthday we were interrupted by a local pastor who recognized me and said, "Aren't you Dr. Leman?" I said I was and he went on, "Oh, I'm so glad I caught you. Today is when I'm supposed to be writing you a note inviting you to talk to our pastors' conference next year on May 16."

He went on to describe the beautiful resort where the conference would be held and how he knew everyone would love to have me come and share with the group.

Krissy had become more and more agitated as the man went on, until finally she poked me in the ribs and said loudly, "My daddy can't come."

"Now wait a minute, Krissy. Daddy and this man are talking. . . ."

The pastor went on with some more of his glorious plans for the conference on May 16 of next year. Krissy could stand it no longer and said even louder, "He can't come!"

Finally I took notice and so did he, and then of course it hit me: May 16 was Krissy's birthday! She was only being very sensitive to Daddy's commitment to *her* day. Fortunately, my pastor friend was wrong about the day he needed me. It turned out to be May 18, so I was able to keep both dates, and my integrity with Krissy. If May 16 had turned out to be the date he needed me, too bad. At our house, May 16 is off limits to the outside world.

Naturally, there are two more inviolate dates on Dr. Leman's calendar each year: November 14 and February 8. After all, Holly and Kevey enjoy choosing where they will eat, what kind of cake they will have, and so on. We are especially big on cakes at our house—rainbow cakes, space cakes, Charlie Brown cakes—*anything is possible on your birthday!*

By speaking up that way to let me know that I couldn't schedule away her special birthday appointment, even when it was a year off, Krissy showed the contradictions you can find in the middle child. A lot of middle children wouldn't have spoken up. They are the kind who resist telling you how they really feel. They are classical avoiders of conflict or confrontation.

But Krissy is sensitive. In many middle children, sensitivity bubbles over into anger. In my counseling, I find that people with anger or hostility are usually first borns or middle borns. It takes a while to flush some of them out because they are pleasers and they may be denying their anger. With Krissy, we always know when she's not happy with something. But with your middle child you may have to dig and probe a bit.

Give your middle child plenty of opportunities to share feelings with you. If you have two middle children, for example, the second and third between a first and a last, keep a close watch on number three, who can really get lost in the shuffle. Don't just make an occasional "How's it going?" remark. Schedule time for a walk or take the child along on an errand and talk in the car. (Talking in a car is a good idea—it's easier to look out the window than right at Mom or Dad when you're trying to share feelings.)

The Squeeze Builds Psychological Muscles

I've made a big point of how social and outgoing middle children may be. Feeling rejected, squeezed, or at least misunderstood at home, they are quicker to go outside the family to make friends.

Parents watch their middle borns come and go and wonder what it is that is so much more attractive about other people's houses. Meanwhile, without realizing it, the middle child is getting invaluable training for life. In making new friends, middle children get practice in committing to relationships and working at keeping them going. They sharpen and refine their social skills as they learn how to deal with the peer group and other people outside the family. When the time to leave home really comes, they are far more ready to deal with the realities of marriage, making a living, and functioning in society.

So, don't despair over your middle child, who always seems to be running off somewhere. In fact, you will be wise to let your middle child know that you understand friends are important. I realize that in some cases the peer group can be a problem, but don't automatically look on the friends as rivals who may lead your child astray. As a rule, try to invite your middle child's friends to your house for an overnight or even a weekend. It's another way to let your middle child know that you think he—and his friends— are very special.

And be aware of one other paradox at work in the middle child's search for friends. While the middle child may feel a little like a fifth wheel at home, home should always remain a lot more safe and forgiving place than the outside world. While the middle child may feel good about all his friends, he can also foul it up with his peer group. When he does, his friends can melt faster than a fudgesicle on the fourth of July in Tucson. That's when he can learn that a squeeze from Mom and Dad isn't so bad after all.

Not all middle children are social lions, of course. Many factors might keep them from having a lot of friends: physical size and appearance, shyness, fears, the need or desire to work or study long hours. But even if the middle child "stays home," so to speak, he still gets automatic training that helps make a better-adjusted person. That training comes in the form of negotiation and compromise.

Middle children can't have it all their own way. The oldest always seems to be getting more, staying up later, staying *out* later, etc. The youngest is getting away with murder and receiving a lot more attention along with it. All this may seem very unfair at the time, but it's great discipline. Middle children are far less likely to be spoiled and therefore they tend to be less frustrated and demanding of life. The typical hassles, irritations, and disappointments of being a middle child are often blessings in disguise.

Recently I talked with a mother who was so

proud of her sixteen-year-old son because he
didn't give her any flack about anything. He was
so unlike so many other teenagers she knew
about—always willing to help, obeying all the
rules, and so on. I smiled and wished her continued success, but I couldn't help wondering if
this kid wasn't really in big trouble. Could he be
bottling things up? Was he the classic pleaser
who would never think of crossing his parents?
What would happen in a few years when the
family umbilical cord was cut and he would be
"out there among 'em"? Would he have the psychological muscles to deal with life?

What am I saying? That all obedient teenagers
are too weak to face life after they leave home?
Not at all. But I am saying that I counsel a lot of
people who were obedient pleasers of Mother
and Dad as they grew up. Now, in adult life,
they're having trouble coping with problems,
neighbors they can't handle, etc., etc. The more
I counsel the more I realize that being squeezed
a little while you're growing up isn't necessarily
all that bad. It's excellent basic training for the
real campaign that starts when you leave home
and strike out on your own.

So, don't despair if you have a middle child
who seems caught in the squeeze right now.
Help him through it, keep his candle lit, and in
the end he may shine brighter than all the rest!

Tips for Parenting the Middle Child

Review the principles of Reality Discipline in chapter 10 and use them in combination with the following suggestions designed especially for use with middle children.

1. Recognize that many middle children are prone to avoid sharing how they really feel about things. If your middle child is an avoider, set aside times for just the two of you to talk. It's important to give this kind of time to every child, but a middle child is least likely to insist on his fair share. Be sure he gets it.

2. Take extra care to make your middle child feel special. Typically, the middle child feels squeezed by the brothers or sisters above and below. The middle child needs those moments when you ask for his opinion, let him choose, etc. One night I took all three of our kids bowling. As we sat down to start our scoresheet, there was an intense discussion over who would roll first. While Holly and Kevey clamored for the honor, I noticed Krissy was not saying a word. I said, "Krissy, you get to choose." So she put down her daddy's name first, then Holly, then Kevey.

3. Along with being sure your middle child feels special, set up some regular privileges he or she can count on having or doing every day or every week. Perhaps it is something as simple

as watching a certain TV program with no interference from others in the family. Maybe it's going to a certain restaurant. The point is, this is the middle child's *exclusive* territory.

4. When was the last time you made a special effort to give your child a new item of clothing rather than a hand-me-down? In some families, income is sufficient so that this is not a problem, but in other homes economics make hand-me-downs a regular part of growing up. An occasional hand-me-down is fine, but your middle child may be particularly appreciative of something new, especially a key item like a coat or a jacket.

5. Listen carefully to your middle child's answers or explanations of what is going on, what they think of certain situations, etc. The desire to avoid conflict and not make waves may get in the way of the real facts. You may have to say, "C'mon now, let's have the whole story. You aren't going to get in trouble. I want to know how you really feel."

6. Above all, be sure the family photo album has its share of pictures of your middle child. Don't let him or her fall victim to the stereotyped fate of seeing thousands of pictures of his older brother or sister and only a few of him!

Chapter Fourteen

Parenting the Last Born: Helping the Family "Cub" Grow Up

My first three words of advice for parents of the last born are: *Beware being manipulated!*

When last born arrives, the real enemy is not that cute little buzzard who marks the end of the family line. *He* can't help being so cute. *She* can't help it if she charms everyone with one toothless smile. The real culprit parents have to battle is well known to Pogo fans, who have met the enemy and realize "he is us."

Remember the three styles of parenting discussed in chapter 10?

Authoritarian parents say, "Do it my way, or else!"

Authoritative parents say, "I'd like to have you do it this way because. . . ."

But permissive parents tell their little last born: "Ahh, you do it your way, you cute little guy."

The Strange Power of the Last Born

Last borns seem to have some strange, mysterious power that softens up parents who have been running a pretty tight ship with the other kids. Maybe the parents have gotten tired; or maybe they've gotten careless because now they think they "know the ropes" and can loosen up. Whatever it is, parents often look the other way when the last born skips chores and drives his older brothers and sisters crazy with pestering, or what I call "setups." (A "setup" is a particular last-born skill which involves bugging an older sibling until he or she lashes out in anger, then running and screaming to Mommy for protection. I was an expert at setting up my brother, Jack.)

If last borns aren't getting away with murder, they are at least trying to manipulate, clown, entertain, and are often likely to be found disturbing somebody's peace.

Even if parents somehow manage to keep the family baby's antics under control, they can still be manipulated by that famous line: "Mommy, I can't do it!" The plaintive cry for help is a great tool last borns use to get parents (as well as older siblings) to snowplow the roads of life for them. They are particularly adept at getting help with schoolwork. I have counseled several children whose seeming helplessness turned their homes into a tutoring establishment right after dishes were done each evening. It's one thing to encourage children with their homework and get them started; it's another to do it for them. A lot of parents get suckered into doing the child's work and believe they are helping the child. Of course they are only hindering the child, because it prohibits him from learning to do his own thinking.

For example, I worked with one seventh-grader whose older brother was in his final year of high school. The parents sent this little redhead to me in the spring of his seventh-grade year because he was doing so poorly in school. The boy was the second and last born of two children.

At first we didn't make much progress. The boy was in all kinds of trouble at school and the parents were going to more conferences than they really wanted to be bothered with. He managed to pass seventh grade, but not by much. We continued working with him throughout the summer and in the fall, big brother went away to college. This seemed to be the breakthrough that was needed. As the boy started into his eighth-grade year, he began responding to some Reality Discipline principles that I had set up, and the parents finally saw some positive results.

The Reality Discipline I asked his parents to use was rather basic:

1. Make the boy stand on his own two feet and not help him with any more of his homework than they absolutely had to.
2. After dinner, no going out to play, no watching television, no doing anything of that nature until responsibilities were taken care of. Responsibilities included chores and certainly schoolwork.
3. No making Mom and Dad tutors for several hours each night. (This went back to making the boy stand on his own two feet.)

This last-born son made an excellent turn-around in the fall of his eighth-grade year. The misbehavior stopped at school and his grades came up nicely without a lot of tutoring by Mom and Dad. The youngster had lived in the shadow of his older brother for so long that he had been completely cowed and discouraged. As I often put it, "His candle had been blown out." The older brother was so confident and competent and so much bigger and stronger that it just left the younger boy wiped out. Once older brother physically left the house, the younger child began to bloom.

And Mom and Dad were relieved when they didn't have to spend three or four hours a night tutoring their last born to keep his grades barely above water. The mother especially was happy because most of the tutoring fell upon her shoulders and she had to work all day to boot. What she had been doing was "setting up school" at 7:00 P.M. and crashing into bed at 11:00 P.M. every night with a tired thirteen-year-old right on her heels. Once the son understood that he had the ability and could do it himself, everything changed.

The Strange Case of Weekend Indigestion

I have also counseled last-born children who just don't care for school. I understand where they are coming from because I felt the same way when I was growing up. Sometimes a child can have real learning problems or disabilities, but in many cases the true issue is attitude.

I'm convinced my disastrous school record could have been greatly improved with one simple step on the part of my parents. My mother should have stopped running down to the school to talk to the counselors. She should have stopped trying to find the cause of little Kevin's problems. If she had simply said, "Hey, kid, no Little League unless you cut it in school," I probably would have turned around by the sixth or seventh grade.

But Mom and Dad never called my bluff. They never drew the line. In a word they were permissive, and I played it for all I could. For example, I had a strange ailment called Friday–

275

Monday Stomachaches. I would wake up on those particular days feeling terrible, and of course, I couldn't go to school. But strangely enough, by midafternoon a miracle had happened. I was instantly healed when the clock struck three! There are other names for my illness. One is "making the weekend longer by faking a stomachache." Somehow my mom never really caught on. I guess she just couldn't believe her little Cub could lie and be in such pain at the same time.

Another trick I mastered was catching "religious fever," particularly on Wednesday or Sunday night when there was work to be done. The dishes would be looming mountainously in the sink and the garbage cans and wastebaskets would be overflowing, but I let none of these mundane temptations keep me from the house of the Lord. "Mom, I've got to get to youth meeting! See you later!" And Mom stayed home and did the work while I did my part to drive the youth leaders crazy.

What or Who Spoils the Last Born?

"Why, the parents do the spoiling, of course," is the answer most people would give. And you're right, but sometimes the parents can get a lot of help from the other children in the family. How spoiled a last born gets can depend on when and where he or she arrives in the family constellation. For example, let's diagram a family consisting of three girls and a last-born boy.

FAMILY A
Female — 11
Female — 9
Female — 6
Male — 3

In this family it looks as if the little guy is totally outnumbered by females. But what can usually occur here is a strong relationship between the mother and the son. After three girls, little Harold will be very precious, especially to Mom, and she is likely to give him the benefit of the doubt when older sisters come and complain about his pestering.

Actually, this family has two last borns, a last-born boy and a last-born girl. This almost guarantees friction between the six-year-old and the three-year-old. In this kind of family, it is very common for "alliances" to form. The way this usually happens in this particular sequence is that the eleven-year-old will form an alliance with the six-year-old and the nine-year-old with the three-year-old.

In many cases, the third-born child in this family could find herself in an unfavorable position. This would be especially true if both of the older girls decided to really mother the little boy and take his side in all of the various arguments and incidents that occur in a family of four. On the other hand, all three of the older girls might decide that the little guy is a pest and be particularly irritated if Mom asks them to do a lot of baby-sitting.

Let's take another look at a family where the last born becomes very special. In this case we have a first-born girl, followed by two boys, and finally along comes "baby princess." The diagram looks like this:

FAMILY B
    Female —   13
    Male   —   12
    Male   —   10
    Female —   4

On the positive side, the last-born girl is in good shape in that she has two older brothers who are likely to wind up becoming her champions, unless she is a total little stinker. With two attentive older brothers, she can grow up learning that men are caring and loving. And with the older sister, she also gets the benefit of more mothering and cuddling, something that first-born girls love to do.

The bad news is that the baby princess can get the idea that the world revolves around her. She may become the apple of Daddy's eye and be able to wrap him around her little finger to get just about anything she wants. If this is carried too far, she can grow up believing she can do this with any man, and be a risky candidate for a happy marriage.

In a word, baby princess could be spoiled rotten unless the parents are aware and careful of not being permissive. She could become snotty, obnoxious, and could become an adult who would make unreasonable demands on just about everyone.

One of the most damaging effects of paternal permissiveness is making things too easy for a child. Later, when the last born has grown to adulthood, he or she may not be prepared for real life. Adversities will be just too much.

I once worked with a family that consisted of a mother (a widow) and five children. There were two older sisters, followed by two older brothers, and then the youngest daughter, who was seven years behind the youngest brother. The father had died when the youngest daughter was thirteen. At the time I counseled the family, the youngest daughter was twenty-six and totally dependent on the mother. For thirteen years the mother and the youngest daughter had virtually lived alone together because the rest of the children had moved out of the house by the time the father had died.

The daughter had been totally protected and "smothered" by her mother to the point that when I saw her, she was uneducated and her confidence was zero. The most challenging tasks she could attempt were housecleaning and baby-sitting.

I realize this is an extreme case of the parent needing the child so badly she didn't allow the child to grow up. But the same thing happens to lesser degrees every time the parent acts permissively and does too much snowplowing of life's roads for a child. When you baby a child too much, you actually render that child useless, or at least cripple him in one way or another.

The Other Side of the Last-Born Coin

One thing I've tried to keep repeating throughout this book is that no birth order fits only one mold. The same characteristics are not always true in every last-born child. You may be a last born who wasn't spoiled that much at all. Or maybe your youngest child is hardly what you would call a manipulator. If anything, your last born is the one being manipulated by the rest of the family. Ironically enough, while youngest children are often coddled and cuddled, they can get more than their share of being cuffed and clobbered, especially by older brothers and sisters.

Birth order specialists claim youngest children have difficulty with "information processing."[1] In other words, they seem to have trouble getting things straight. The older kids always seem to be so smart—so authoritative and knowing. No matter that the older kids are often totally incorrect in their dogmatic pronouncements to the baby of the family—the baby *perceives* they are right because they are so much bigger, stronger, and "smarter."

As a last born, I can remember feeling plenty stupid when Sally or Jack would set me straight on anything from the facts of life to the time of day. My big brother, Jack—five years older—had a very direct approach for setting me straight. He'd belt me one.

Of course, I often had it coming. I was a pro at setting up Jack by goading and pestering him until he'd lose his cool and hit me. Then I'd scream bloody murder and Dad would get on his case. It was great fun, but there was a high price tag. Sooner or later Jack would get me alone where I couldn't frame him or convince my parents that it was all his fault. Of course he never really killed me. He just pounded me a little for the sake of general principles.

In one case, he had a different approach to setting me straight. He became informer and turned me in for smoking cigarettes at age eight behind the chicken coop. That one really cost me. I had to go straight to bed with no dinner, pretty tough treatment for the baby Cub, who usually got away with murder.

Sally set little Kevin straight in another way.

As my "second mother" she often became distressed when I was too coarse, too loud, or just plain too smart-mouthed. But she had a different style. She had a way of making me feel as if I wanted to do better. She wouldn't say, "Don't behave like that," or "What's the matter with you, why don't you shape up?"

Whenever anyone—parents, teachers, etc.—told me not to do something with that tone of voice, it was just like pouring gasoline on a fire. It only goaded me on to do more things to get attention by bucking the establishment.

But Sally had a different approach. Actually she was something of a master amateur psychologist. When I acted up, she would often say things such as, "Do you really want to act like that?"

I'd try to be cute and respond, "Sure I do—that's what makes it fun." But deep inside I knew different. Sally was already planting seeds to be watered by my math teacher when I was in high school and carefully cultivated by a beautiful nurse's aide whom I would meet while doing janitor duties in the Tucson Medical Center.

Of course, in all fairness to the memory of my past, there were times when I could get to Sally just as easily as I got to Jack. I remember her screaming, "Mother, would you get him *out* of here?" And she frequently complained, "He gets away with murder—you never let me do that when I was his age."

Recap on Why Last Borns Have No Bed of Roses

With all of their legendary "easy street" existence and their reputation for "getting away with murder," last borns face several bumps in life that belie the claim that they have it made. We've already looked at two major ones. First, last borns may become too dependent and stay babies if they are coddled and cuddled too much. Everyone and anyone in the family may be guilty of this, from the parents to the older brothers and sisters.

The other major problem that we've looked at is that last borns can take a lot of abuse, pressure, resentment, and teasing from older brothers and sisters. Parents may sometimes think they need a crystal ball—or maybe a new piece of wonder software for the computer—to help them figure out when the baby of the family is really getting it in the neck or when he is just working his manipulative wiles. When counseling parents of last borns, I usually tell them if they must err, let it be on the side of helping the baby of the family stand on his own two feet and cope, even if it means getting teased or intimidated on occasion.

A lot depends on age and size differences. After all, when you're the baby cub, getting teased is one thing, getting trampled is another. At our house, Kevey enjoys substantial protection from

Mom and Dad because he's only seven while his sisters are eleven and twelve and a lot bigger. Of course, Kevey can really push and pester at times and there are moments when he ventures out to the brink of disaster. Then I get his attention by saying, "Kevey, if you don't shape up, in three seconds I'm going to turn those two sisters loose." Kevey shapes up—and fast. Krissy, especially, strikes fear in his heart. She is strong, quick, and when it comes to little brothers who are pests, not too patient.

One other hurdle for last borns is well worth underlining. Because they are last, nothing they do is really original. Their older brothers or sisters have already learned to talk, read, tie shoes, and ride a bike. And, let's face it. It *is* hard for Mom or Dad to get excited about the third or fourth lopsided pencil holder or paperweight to be brought home from school art class in the last five or ten years.

Family specialist Edith Neisser catches the spirit of frustration last borns often feel because nothing they do seems to be very big news. She quotes an eighth-grader who had this to say about having older brothers and sisters:

> No matter what I ever do, it won't be important. When I graduate from high school, they'll be graduating from college or getting married; then if I ever do get through with college, Sis will probably be

having a baby. Why, even when I die it won't be anything new to my family; nobody will even be here to pay any attention.[2]

If you have any junior highs in your home, you may have heard the same kind of exaggerated dramatics, but there is a kernel of real truth in what this girl said. The key phrase is "Nobody will even be here to pay any attention." That is something every parent can be aware of with the last born: "Am I paying enough attention to little Harold's 'firsts' in life? Yes, it's my third or fourth paperweight but it's only his *first*. I should make as big a deal out of *his* firsts as anyone else's."

At least be assured that your last born is well aware of his special slot in the family. It's not likely he wants to trade. This all came home to me in living color as I was driving alone with Kevey recently. Just for fun, I asked him, "How about it, Kevey? Would you mind if Mommy had another baby?"

There was a long pause as Kevey gave the question serious consideration. Finally he said, "I guess it's okay—just as long as she's a girl!"

Tips for Parenting the Last-Born Child

Using Reality Discipline is especially critical with the family baby because of the natural tendency to ease up and slack off. Be sure to see chapter 10, especially the principles regarding accountability and responsibility. In addition, try the suggestions below.

1. Be sure your last born has his fair share of responsibilities around the house. Last borns often wind up with very little to do for two reasons: (A) they are masters at ducking out of the work that needs to be done; (B) they are so little and "helpless," the rest of the family members decide it's easier to do it themselves.

2. Along the same lines, be sure your last born does not get away with murder in regard to family rules and regulations. Statistics show the last born is least likely to be disciplined and the least likely to have to toe the mark the way the older children did. It wouldn't hurt to make notes on how you held the older kids responsible and enforce the same bedtime and other rules on your last born.

3. While you're making sure you don't coddle your youngest child, don't let him get clobbered or lost in the shuffle, either. Last borns are well known for feeling that "nothing I do is important." Make a big deal out of your last born's accomplishments and be sure he or she gets a

fair share of "marquee time" on the refrigerator door with his school papers, drawings, etc.

4. Introduce your youngest child to reading very early. Six months is not too young to start reading to your child with brightly colored illustrated books. When your child starts reading, don't do the work for him. Last borns tend to "like to be read to" and will let you do most of the work if they can get away with it. This may be one of the reasons last borns are well known for being the poorest readers in their families.

5. Whenever necessary, call baby's bluff. I have always felt my parents should have cracked down on me regarding school when I was young. But they never really put on the pressure. They never gave me choices like, "Shape up at school or drop Little League," or "No homework, no television programs tonight."

6. Try to get your last born's baby book completed before he or she is twenty-one. Life seems to pile up on parents with the arrival of the third and fourth child. Check to see if you're neglecting the last born because you just don't seem to have as much time as you used to. Let other things go if necessary to be sure you provide time for each child.

7. Oh, yes—along the way, try to pick out a nice first born for your last born to marry. The odds are high they'll make a great team!

Epilogue

The One Thing You Can't Do Without

If you've gotten this far, you are probably a first born who will enjoy reviewing key points. If you are an intrepid middle child or last born, hang in there. I have one more story I think you'll like. First, the key points to remember about birth order:

1. As important as a child's order of birth may be, it is only an influence, not a final fact of life forever set in cement and unchangeable as far as how that child will turn out.
2. The way parents treat their children is equally important to their birth order, environment, physical and mental characteristics.
3. Every birth order has inherent strengths and weaknesses. Parents must accept both while helping the child develop positive traits and cope with negative ones.
4. No birth order is "better" or more desirable than another. First borns seem to have

a corner on achievement and the headlines, but the door is wide open for later borns to make their mark. It is up to them.

5. Birth order information does not give the total psychological picture for anyone. No system of personality development can do that. Birth order statistics and characteristics are indicators that combine with physical, mental, and emotional factors to give the bigger picture.

6. Understanding some basic principles of birth order is not a formula for automatically solving problems or changing your personality overnight. Changing oneself is the hardest task any human being can attempt; it takes long, hard work.

Only One Thing Is Absolutely Necessary

After spending thousands of hours preparing to be a psychologist and therapist and then thousands more talking with people from every walk of life and every kind of situation, I realize you can never know too much. At the same time, after you read all the books, use all the techniques, and say all the right words (you hope), there is only one thing you dare not try to get along without. This secret weapon works equally well with any birth order. But without it, family living in particular becomes a hopeless task.

The following little story describes this most necessary parenting skill. In a way, I'm not talking about something you learn in so many lessons, like operating a word processor or driving a car. I speak of an art that you acquire slowly and sometimes painfully. And just about the time you think you are getting the hang of it, something happens to remind you of how basic life is and how far you still have to go.

The spring Holly was ten, one day I decided I needed to brush up on one of the parental activities I had advocated so enthusiastically in a new book I had just finished called *Making Children Mind Without Losing Yours.* The activity? Spend more one-on-one time with each child. Combining a full load of counseling appointments with trying to travel, appear on talk shows, and promote books on better parenting is a good way to become a physician who needs a dose of his own medicine.

Holly was on my mind and available, so I called Sande and told her I thought it was time to spend a one-on-one evening with our first born. Sande was all for it.

I kept my plan a secret until after work, when I picked up Holly after her bobby-sox softball game. As she got in the car, I said, "Holly, how would you like to go out with Daddy tonight?"

Her first words were, "Without *them?*"

"Just the two of us."

"ALL RIGHT!"

Holly tossed her glove in the backseat and we took off to what was indeed a great evening. We pulled in the driveway at 10:30 P.M., well past curfew for a ten-year-old on a Thursday night with school coming up the next morning.

As I turned off the ignition, Holly asked a question. In retrospect, I now realize it was a very significant one. My assertive little first born had really enjoyed her evening without *them*. Now she wanted a little icing on her cake, just for the sake of general principles.

"Daddy, for a special treat, can I pull my sleeping bag into your room and sleep on the floor next to your bed?"

As the world's leading advocate of Reality Discipline, I immediately realized I must act swiftly. After all, I know what is best for my kids. Faster than any family expert should, I replied, "Holly, no. Now listen, it's late and it's a school night. I want you to go to bed—you need a *good night's sleep.*"

Before "good night's sleep" passed my lips, I realized I had violated one of the principles I teach in counseling, seminars, and my books. *Don't always give an immediate response to a child's request.* Think about it for a few seconds at least, and try to give the child an answer that has understanding and reason behind it.

Actually, my snap answer contained excellent

logic—for an adult. It *was* a school night, it *was* late, and Holly *did* need her sleep. Of course, I needed mine as well, because I was due up at 5:00 A.M. to catch a 7:00 A.M. plane to appear at a sales conference being held by my publisher in New Jersey, where I would extol the wisdom of my forthcoming book *Making Children Mind Without Losing Yours.*

Holly was not impressed by my fatherly advice and wisdom about a "good night's sleep." She planned a good night's sleep—next to my bed. I was being unreasonable, and immediately the tears trickled down her first-born cheeks.

"But Daddy, I just want to sleep by your bed . . ."

I should have remembered that Holly is more of a powerful perfectionist than a mild-mannered pleaser. But I was tired—it was late and I had to be up early.

"Holly, no. The floor is hard. You won't sleep all that well. Now, come on—we've had a great evening together. Don't spoil it!"

For Holly everything was already spoiled. "You never let me do *anything!*" she wailed, as the wonderful evening blew up in my face.

I got Holly into the house and into bed, still sobbing, "You never let me do anything, you never let me do anything."

Feeling frustrated, angry, and guilty all at once, I decided I had better finish packing— there wouldn't be much time at five o'clock in the morning. I had asked Sande to wash and iron a pair of slacks and a shirt I wanted to wear on the plane. Sure enough, my loving wife had washed them. She had even dried them, and as I learned later, had then forgotten all about ironing them and had gone to bed.

Picture the scene: I could hear Holly still sniffing and sobbing and mumbling, "You never let me do anything." It was getting toward midnight. I had to catch a plane at the crack of dawn, and I was standing at the ironing board considering options:

A. wearing something else (but this was a favorite combination and comfortable for the plane ride)

B. getting Sande up to do it (bad idea, she takes forty minutes minimum to wake up once she's fallen asleep)

C. doing it myself (maybe I could use it when I spoke at the publisher's sales conference as an illustration of what a loving and sacrificial husband I am)

But Holly's wailing kept distracting me. She wouldn't stop. If anything, it was getting louder. *She's being a powerful little buzzard, Leman,* I told myself. *Time to pull the rug!*

I stalked into Holly's room and made my speech. Actually it was more of a shouted tirade:

"All right, Holly, now listen up! I've had enough of this, do you understand me? We had a wonderful evening—wonderful. And now it's time for you to be in bed and asleep and you know why I'm upset, Holly? Because I just went out there and found my clothes that your mother was supposed to have ready for me in a wrinkled mess, and *I'm not in a real good mood!*"

I capped my screaming and yelling by telling her she was going to bed and that was *final!*

I came out of Holly's room, slammed the door, shook the whole house, and woke everybody up—well, Sande sort of rolled over. I went into the family room and turned on the late news. I sat there trying to get hold of myself, and then the "guilties" really got to me. I knew I was wrong. I had overreacted, to say the least. Holly's cries had subsided but I knew I had to do something to make it right. I wanted to give her a kiss. Maybe she was asleep, but I still needed to give her a kiss.

I pulled myself together and, feeling terrible, gently pushed open Holly's door.

Holly wasn't in her bed.

Now she's disobeyed me. I'm going to kill her!

I went tearing through the house, looking for Holly. What was it I had just written in *Making Children Mind* . . . about using spanking sparingly? Well *this time* I had a few good swats to spare, all right. My first guess was our bedroom. Holly had probably sneaked into bed with her mother or was lying on the floor in that sleeping bag, just as she wanted to do in the first place.

But Holly wasn't in our bedroom. So I checked Kevey's room—no Holly. I checked Krissy's room—still no Holly. My ten-year-old didn't seem to be in the house and it was after eleven o'clock at night. Had she run away?

Whenever I get anxious I do what any trained therapist does to get himself together. I go right to the refrigerator to eat. On my way to the kitchen I walked by the sewing room and there was Holly, ironing one of my shirts.

Her first words were sort of cute when you think about the first born and perfectionism: "Daddy, I don't iron real good."

Holly was trying her best, and using the old-fashioned method for sprinkling the shirt—her tears.

I just said, "Oh, Holly, would you forgive me?"

And Holly said, "I've ruined the whole evening . . . I've ruined the whole evening."

"No, Holly, Daddy ruined the whole evening. I was wrong. Will you forgive me?"

One thing about Holly, she loves emphasis: "I've ruined the whole evening . . . I've ruined the whole evening."

I tried again. "Holly, will you hush up and let me apologize?"

Holly put down the iron, walked two steps, and burrowed her head in my chest. She squeezed me, hugged me, held me, and told me she loved me. I did the same. One hundred twenty seconds later, Holly was in her bed, fast asleep.

Somehow I got the ironing done. Somehow I caught the plane the next morning with only a few hours' sleep. I arrived at the publishing house and presented my new book on parenting to the sales staff. I didn't tell them about the bumbling and stumbling I had done just a few hours before, but the easiest part of my presentation was when I said:

"I believe the time we really look big in a child's eyes is when we go to them to apologize for our mistakes, not theirs. I believe the words no parent can do without are *I was wrong. Will you forgive me?*"

Source Notes

Chapter 1

1. See "Using Birth Order and Sibling Dynamics in Career Counseling," Richard W. Bradley, *The Personnel and Guidance Journal,* September 1982, p. 25. Bradley quotes from the article "Is First Best?" in *Newsweek,* January 6, 1969, p. 37.

2. See the article "Motivational and Achievement Differences Among Children of Various Ordinal Birth Positions," R. L. Adams and B. N. Phillips, *Child Development,* March 1972, p. 157.

3. See Walter Toman, *Family Constellation* (New York: Springer Publishing Company, 1976), p. 33.

Chapter 2

1. Dr. James Dobson, *Hide or Seek* (Old Tappan: Fleming H. Revell Company, 1974). See especially chapter 2.

2. See Bradford Wilson and George Edington, *First Child, Second Child* (New York: McGraw-Hill Book Company, 1981), p. 259.

3. According to Wilson and Edington, *First Child, Second Child,* a woman of forty is three to four times more likely to produce twins than someone half her age. Also, women usually give birth at least one time before they have twins. Twins usually grow up with at least one older sibling, and their parents are often near forty or older when they are born (see p. 262).

4. See Psalms 139:13–16.

5. See James H. S. Bossard, *The Large Family System* (Philadelphia: University of Pennsylvania Press, 1966), p. 79.
6. See Walter Toman, *The Family Constellation* (New York: Springer Publishing Company, Third Edition, 1976), p. 5.
7. See, for example, Romans 1:16.

Chapter 3
1. The story about Sande and the undone salmon also appears in my book *Sex Begins in the Kitchen* (Ventura, California: Regal Books, 1981), p. 61, but I repeat it here with a few embellishments because it so clearly illustrates the compliant first born who would rather please than protest or complain.
2. See Genesis 4:3–8.
3. "What Scholars, Strippers, and Congressmen Share," study by Richard Zweigenhaft, reported by Jack Horn, *Psychology Today,* May 1976, p. 34.

Chapter 4
1. "Does the Only Child Grow Up Miserable?" Toni Falbo, *Psychology Today,* May 1976, p. 60.
2. Alfred Adler, *Understanding Human Nature* (New York: Fawcett World Library, 1969), p. 127.
3. See Lucille K. Forer, Ph.D., with Henry Still, *The Birth Order Factor* (New York: David McKay Company, Inc., 1976), pp. 9, 10.
4. See Forer, *Birth Order Factor,* p. 255.

Chapter 5
1. See Bradford Wilson and George Edington, *First Child, Second Child* (New York: McGraw-Hill Book Company, 1981), p. 29.
2. Adapted from Dr. David Stoop, *Self-Talk: Key to Personal Growth* (Old Tappan, New Jersey: Fleming H. Revell Company, 1982), p. 120.

Chapter 6
1. See Bradford Wilson and George Edington, *First Child, Second Child* (New York: McGraw-Hill Book Company, 1981), p. 92.
2. This is quoted in Edith G. Neisser, *Brothers and Sisters* (New York: Harper and Brothers, 1951), p. 154. From *The Middle Moffat* by Eleanor Estes.
3. See Wilson and Edington, *First Child,* p. 95.
4. See Wilson and Edington, *First Child,* p. 99.
5. See Wilson and Edington, *First Child,* p. 99.
6. See Wilson and Edington, *First Child,* p. 102.
7. See Wilson and Edington, *First Child,* p. 104.
8. See Wilson and Edington, *First Child,* p. 103.
9. See "Birth Order and Relationships," Pam Hait, *Sunday Woman,* September 12, 1982, p. 4.

Chapter 7
1. See Bradford Wilson and George Edington, *First Child, Second Child* (New York: McGraw-Hill Book Company, 1981), p. 108.
2. See "A Lastborn Speaks Out—At Last," Mopsy Strange Kennedy, *Newsweek,* November 7, 1977, p. 22.
3. See Wilson and Edington, *First Child,* p. 108.
4. See also my book *Parenthood Without Hassles* (Eugene, Oregon: Harvest House Publishers, 1979), p. 11.
5. See also my book *Parenthood Without Hassles,* p. 12.
6. Matthew 18:21, 22.
7. See Wilson and Edington, *First Child,* pp. 109, 110.

Chapter 8
1. Walter Toman, *Family Constellation* (New York: Springer Publishing Company, 1976).

Chapter 9
1. Alfred Adler, *The Practice and Theory of Individual Psychology* (Totowa, New Jersey: Littlefield, Adams & Company, 1968), p. 3.
2. See Adler, *Practice and Theory,* p. 3.

Chapter 10
1. See Kevin Leman, *Making Children Mind Without Losing Yours* (Old Tappan, New Jersey: Fleming H. Revell Company, 1984), p. 11.
2. See Leman, *Making Children Mind,* p. 27.
3. See Leman, *Making Children Mind,* pp. 27, 28.
4. See Leman, *Making Children Mind,* p. 109.
5. See Leman, *Making Children Mind,* pp. 88, 89.
6. See Leman, *Making Children Mind,* pp. 115, 116.

Chapter 11
1. See Luke 15:11–32.

Chapter 12
1. Genesis 25:19–34; 27:1–40.

Chapter 14
1. See Bradford Wilson and George Edington, *First Child, Second Child* (New York: McGraw-Hill Book Company, 1981), pp. 110, 111.
2. See Edith G. Neisser, *Brothers and Sisters* (New York: Harper and Brothers, 1951), pp. 165, 166.

Other Publications by Dr. Kevin Leman

   A Child's Ten Commandments to Parents
   Parenthood Without Hassles—Well, Almost
   Sex Begins in the Kitchen
   Smart Girls Don't, and Guys Don't Either

Other Family and Child-Rearing Resources by Dr. Kevin Leman

Video Series
   Growing Up Whole in a Breaking Up World
   Love 'Em and Keep 'Em: The Challenge of Raising Kids
   Sex and the Christian Family
Video series available for rental/purchase from
   Covenant Video
   3200 W. Foster Avenue
   Chicago, Illinois 60625
   1-800-621-1290
Film Series
   Growing Up Whole in a Breaking Down World
Film series distributed by
   Gospel Films
   Box 455
   Muskegon, Michigan 49443
   1-800-253-0413
Audio Series
   Parenthood Without Hassles—Well, Almost
   Success Motivation Institute, Inc.
   Waco, Texas
   Creating Intimacy in Marriage
   Vision House
   Ventura, California

Growing up Whole in a Breaking Down World
Way to Grow Series
Word, Inc.
Waco, Texas
Language of Listening
Word, Inc.
Waco, Texas

For information regarding speaking engagements or seminars, write or call:

Dr. Kevin Leman
1325 N. Wilmot Rd.
Suite 320
Tucson, Arizona 85712
602-886-9925